One Heart – One Life

with
compliments
Rohan

One Heart – One Life

The scientific guide to complete mind-body renewal for healthy living and dynamic vitality

S. Rohan Jayasinghe MD, MSpM, FRACP
Specialist Cardiologist/ Sports Physician- New York

Revere Life Publishing

Disclaimer

This book is intended to be a source of general health related knowledge only. This is not a treatment guide or a therapeutic manual. For all your health related matters you should seek the advice and services of a qualified medical practitioner at all times. The information may change according to new scientific discoveries being made in the areas of medicine and clinical sciences. The facts contained in this book are as accurate as the contemporary knowledge at the time of publication. The case vignettes in this book resemble common and typical real life events in contemporary cardiology practice and in no way relates to any individual alive or deceased. The names and events mentioned in the case vignettes are completely imaginary and does not relate or refer to any individual alive or deceased.

ISBN#: 0-615-12590-5

First published June 2004

Printed in New York, United States of America

Cover design and photography (copyright) – Jill Gregory

Revere Life Publishing – New York. Sydney
reverelifepublishing@yahoo.com

To Lisa with love ....

Preface

Good health is what we all desire. But often we take health for granted. As I have observed in my medical practice, good health is not a privilege but a choice. It is the choices that we make in our everyday life that eventually decide the course our health takes in the present time and in the future. That is why a group of common diseases including heart disease have been identified as lifestyle disorders. Your heart is like no other organ in your body. You only get one chance with your heart. Any damage done to your heart is irreversible and permanent. But the interesting truth us that on most instances you have the complete authority to make the right choices to protect your heart and to prevent heart disease.

There is much talk about mind-body medicine. The main advocates of this concept however have been the practitioners of alternative therapeutics. Your conventional doctors very often focus exclusively on the physical attributes of health and illness. In this book I interpret the scientific validity of the concept of mind-body medicine and explain how it fundamentally and directly relates to conventional "western" medicine. I also explain in the chapters to come how your mind and your body become one single entity in form and function and how the mind factors affect your physical health and how your body factors affect your mental health. The main theme of this book is to put right your mind factors and your body factors to generate health, particularly your heart health.

One of the three keys to the wholesome mind factor that I discuss in this book is acquisition of knowledge. I teach many things that you should know about your heart. These include factors related to the health of your heart, extensive facts about heart disease, its treatment and very importantly its prevention. In the pages to come you will learn how heart disease evolved in our society to become the most important public health problem of modern era and how treatment methods of current day progressed from its rudimentary levels. The scientific and historical facts included in this book will enhance your knowledge to empower you to make you fully capable of making the right decisions in regards to healthy living as well as the right therapy in situations of illness.

For the most part the pioneering giants of conventional (western) medicine ignored the pearls of ancient wisdom from the east in their study of heart disease, its prevention and its treatment. However since of late these valuable truths are being exposed and introduced to the mainstream but still at far lesser levels than desired. In the chapters to come I introduce to you the scientifically proven benefits of traditional eastern medical concepts, its philosophy and practice. Extensive discussions and teachings on yoga, Tai Chi and even novel forms of physical practices such as Pilates contained in the pages of this book will make your knowledge broad and well rounded.

You will find many simple and easy-to-follow practical instructions on diet, exercise and simple choices of day-to-day life that matters to your health. You will learn why sex is so important to your health. You will learn the principles of diet watching, to optimize the health value of the food you eat without compromising the taste and the variety of your meals. I introduce the revolutionary new diet that I call the "Life Diet" that is based on the scientifically proven health concepts and the results of powerful and convincing clinical research. The principles on which this diet is designed has proven efficacy to cause weight loss, maintain weight control, bring about good health and give longevity. In the pages of this book are some very practical and scientifically sound secrets to living your life to the max- tips on how to enjoy life to the full and yet be robustly healthy and youthful.

The scientific concepts and information in this book are cutting edge and most modern. I have endeavored to include all the latest knowledge on everything relevant to the theme of this book with objective judgment and impartial interpretation.

This book is all about putting things right with your life from the simple act of breathing to choosing the best way to treat your heart if you have heart disease. At the end of reading this you will know how to create the right balance between your mind and body factors to make you feel and be the best everyday of your life. Remember it is your choice. To make the right choices you need the right knowledge. This book is the "knowledge prescription' that will generate the power within you to make the right choices everyday and at all times.

I wish to thank my parents, my grandfather and Lisa for constant support and encouragement during the writing of this book. Lisa, thank you for lending me time. I specially thank my late grandfather Mr.WA Sangadasa, a man of great wisdom, for teaching me some important concepts of traditional eastern health practice and philosophy.

S Rohan Jayasinghe MD, MSpM, FRACP
jayasinghe@medscape.com

New York, New York
Spring 2004

Contents

Foreword

It gives me great pleasure to write the foreword to this timely book written by Dr Rohan Jayasinghe titled One Heart One Life. Heart disease is the biggest killer in our society. The high prevalence of heart disease is fundamentally due to the general and wide spread ignorance about important matters related to heart health in our society. This book is an apt attempt at delivering that essential yet relatively untapped knowledge on how to get healthy out to the public. The great expectation of attempts such as this book is eventually to create increased public awareness and a psychology of inquiry to facilitate improved health and general well being among the members of our society.

Medical technology is advancing fast. Everyday new diagnostic and treatment methods are being introduced and made available to the public. This is more so with cardiology, in particular interventional cardiology in that the way heart disease is addressed and managed seems to change dramatically over short intervals of time. Due to this rapid advancement of knowledge and technology, an ever-widening gap seems to be developing between what the medical world and the doctors know and what the general public and therefore the patient population knows. This book makes a fine attempt at bridging this gap by introducing and reviewing the latest in the diagnostics and therapeutics used in the contemporary practice of cardiology.

Dr Jayasinghe has done a fine job in transforming the factual matter in this book to interesting reading material by incorporating very dramatic case scenarios that depict how modern cardiology is practiced. The discussions on the prevention of cardiac disease and promotion of health are invaluable sources of essential knowledge. The topics and concepts discussed and the healthy living plans introduced are scientifically sound and based on published research.

This book provides fine reading material that is both educational and entertaining. One Heart and One Life can be recommended as essential reading.

Dr David Brown MD
Director of Interventional Cardiology
Beth Israel Medical Center
New York, New York

Chapter 1

If only he knew

I was by my self, waiting for a flight at the Los Angeles airport one summer afternoon. The wait for my trans-pacific flight seemed too long. Few options in hand to kill time included reading, people watching, napping or settling for a drink. I was sipping an espresso seated at the coffee bar on the second floor when I captured the glimpse of a young family that approached the table next to mine. It was a happy family with two angelic little girls. One girl appeared to be about 5 years old and her sister about 3. First the two adorable little girls came running to the table and clambered onto two chairs. They were giggling and laughing – seemingly very excited about some thing. Soon their mother followed through. She was a charming woman, who was obviously pregnant. Next came the father. He appeared to be in his mid thirties. A seemingly nice man who appeared to adore and love his family. Though he looked the rough type, his display of affection to his little family exposed a very delicate personality. He was heavy set – essentially obese. He had a prominent abdominal bulge. I could surmise beyond any doubt that he was a smoker- the fat packet of cigarettes in his shirt pocket was a giveaway.

He was carrying in his arms a meal that he had just purchased for his family. That may be one reason that the two little girls appeared so very excited. He had paper bags full of ham burghers, cheese burghers, French fries and a family size sweet chocolate dessert. I felt a sudden sense of sadness upon seeing the picture unfolding before me. Here was a young man with a pregnant wife, two adorable little kids and his whole life ahead of him. It was clear to me that this man would not remain healthy for too long. He may not even live for too long. He was in a highway to a heart attack. He had a dangerous combination of coronary risk factors that would one day not to far away, cause a massive heart attack and either kill him or disable him for life.

He was obese, apparently smoked, ate unhealthy food, belonged to a high risk socioeconomic group and I could bet that he had high cholesterol levels, high blood pressure and possibly diabetes or early diabetes too. He was male. His blood pressure ought to be high given his body weight. Why was he going on with his unhealthy life style putting at stake all that he should live for? There was one reason - Lack of knowledge-a deadly ignorance! And he is not alone! This is the case with millions who are at risk of heart disease in our society. A deadly condition that can be avoided by making some simple changes to your life style.

Education and acquisition of knowledge are the only ways out of this dire fate. Every one in our society is at risk. Heart disease is a major problem in our society. Acquiring some basic knowledge about this organ that sustains your life and about the common diseases that can consume it, and together with i your life is of critical importance. In this book I endeavor to share with you how the way you live decides the fate of your heart and your life and how best to optimize your life style to protect your heart and your life. I also discuss how cutting-edge modern science and pearls of ancient wisdom combined together can give you the best chance of saving your heart and your life.

Saving hearts, treating people

The excitement in the air was tangible. For an outside observer the whole episode may appear utterly chaotic and confusing. I was donning my blue scrubs as my assistant who had scrubbed ahead of me was preparing the operating table. There were nurses running up and down opening up sterile equipment kits for my assistant. He picked up each equipment carefully, prepared and laid down on the sterile table in a very orderly manner so as to avoid any confusion during the often fast-phase and very delicate operation that we were gearing up for. There were other nurses rushing in and drawing up essential drugs. The lab technician was wheeling in the different machines that would be necessary for this life saving procedure. He would plug in and keep all machines ready to avoid any delays in delivering treatment. A delay of few seconds may mean the loss of life and we all were gravely aware of this crucial fact. Next to the sterile equipment table was the empty operating table still waiting for the patient. Within the matter of a few minutes the cardiac catheterization laboratory was ready for the operation and a relative lull descends. I put on my sterile gloves as the buzz was re-ignited with the wheeling in of the patient. The noise from the radio communication equipment of the medical emergency team and the continuous beeping of the patient's EKG monitor helped only to add to the clamor that seemed to build up again.

Through the gaps between the people who were transferring the patient to the table I could see the EKG monitor hooked on to the patient. The moving brilliant green lines of the EKG waves reconfirmed to me first hand the gravity of the situation that I had already been impressed upon by the doctors in the emergency room. The EKG waveform he had is nick named the "tomb stone" wave pattern in the cardiac circles. It is called so because each heart wave resembles the shape of a tombstone and usually such a pattern suggests a massive heart attack due to the total blockage of a large coronary artery. Wide spread tomb stone waves indicated to me that this man was having a major-life threatening heart attack involving a large area of his heart. His life was literally hanging on a thread.

Then I saw his face. It was a young man-possibly in his mid thirties. His eyes were sunken and the face pale- with an unmistakable expression of agony. Covering his nose was the oxygen mask with jets of vapor rising from its side-holes. As I was watching the regular green waveform of the EKG monitor, suddenly it became irregular and chaotic. Its periodic beep turned into an irritating continuous alarm. The patient went into cardiac arrest right before our eyes.

Another doctor from the cardiology team grabbed the defibrillator pads in a flash and placed on the bare chest of the young man and shouted "hands off the table". Next moment the patient jerked with his back arching upward and all four of his limbs stiffening straight as the high voltage electric shock was delivered to his chest. In an instant all eyes turned to the EKG monitor anticipating the restoration of the regular rhythm, which would essentially mean restoration of life. But after the massive spike denoting the delivered shock the rhythm remained unchanged and chaotic.

"Still in VF….shocking again" shouted the doctor with the defibrillator pads in his hands. The few seconds wait for the defibrillator to re-charge felt like eternity. Meanwhile the patient was kept alive by ventilating with a self-inflating resuscitation bag. Another person was giving the cardiac massage with his fists placed on the patient's bare chest. The second shock was delivered and the rhythm restored. There was a sigh of relief. "Start adrenaline and clear the table" I shouted. I was desperate to start the intervention to open his blocked coronary. If I did not get in there and open the artery immediately the patient was destined to die very soon. It was a deadly race against time. Time was crucial as any delays could certainly mean loss of life.

I drew up the local anesthetic agent lidocaine to a syringe and approached the patient's groin with my scalpel and the 6 French gauge needle. My assisting doctor had sterilized the operating field and covered the patient with blue sterile drapes. I hurriedly established access to the big artery supplying the patient's leg. Next moment we fed a long hollow tube called a "catheter" towards his heart. First we engaged and visualized the coronary artery supplying the right side of the heart. It was clearly normal. We knew that the block was in the left sided coronary artery since the EKG was showing changes in the front wall of the heart. Next we engaged the left coronary artery with a different catheter and injected the x-ray contrast die. Right in front of our eyes the black and white x-ray television monitor flashed the dreaded and unmistakable "widow maker" sign- a tight block in the large artery that supplies blood to the all-important front wall of the heart. Front wall of the heart has the most amount of muscle that helps pump blood all over the body. Death of heart muscle in this region –if large enough- is not compatible with life. Even if the patient were to survive, the damage done would be so devastating that he or she would suffer a slow death from cardiac failure – unless treated with heart transplantation. But our patient would be lucky to escape alive with minimal damage if we could unblock the artery quickly enough. So the next moment all efforts were concentrated on one thing – demolishing the widow maker.

We formulated our strategy of operation while hurriedly preparing for the next phase of the intervention. We quickly inserted a wire into the right side chamber of the heart to externally stimulate the heart with electrical impulses if in case it were to stop beating during the procedure. A larger catheter was introduced to the left coronary artery. Blood-thinning medication heparin was administered to the patient and a hi-tech catheter device was introduced to the coronary artery to extract the blood clot that was blocking it. This process is called thrombectomy – or removal of the clot. The special catheter acts like a vacuum cleaner and extracts the big blood clot blocking the coronary, thus unblocking the artery and restoring the blood flow. Once the clot was removed we could appreciate good blood flow to the heart muscle. Instantaneously the EKG waveform flipped back to the normal pattern. In the following angiogram we could see an ulcer and a cholesterol plaque at the spot in the coronary artery where the clot stood before its extraction. We decided to unblock the artery further by introducing and inflating a miniature balloon to where it was blocked- a process called "angioplasty". Subsequently we sealed the ulcer with a precisely sized slotted metal coil called a "stent". The operation was a success. Patient's heart appeared to function well once again. And he was maintaining a good blood pressure. His life was safe-at least for the time being.

As I was coming out of the catheterization room, we get another call from ER – another patient having a heart attack has been brought in. This time the patient was a little older. After listening to the story I decided that the best treatment for this patient too would be urgent coronary intervention to unblock the coronary artery that was causing the heart attack. "Bring him on" I responded and hurriedly proceeded to the adjoining catheterization room that was being prepared. Few minutes later the patient was wheeled in and the whole cycle repeats. We unblocked the coronary artery and the patient lives to see another day. This is a brief vignette of the usual sequence of events that takes place in the many thousand cath-labs of busy hospitals all over the country everyday.

Few hours later, after finishing the second operation, I met the first patient we treated in the recovery lounge. I will call him Tom. He was 35 years old, a police officer with a young family. His wife was 30 years and he had two sons aged 4 years and 5 years. He had a strong family history of early heart attacks with his father suffering a heart attack at 40 and his brother at 37. He smoked. This story alone was enough to explain the risk he was at. But interestingly he was totally unaware of his high coronary risk. "If I only knew doc" he sighed during the course of our discussion. Tom is extremely lucky that medical science has advanced so much that he could literally be snatched back from the jaws of death with the delivery of appropriate treatment quite promptly. Furthermore with the help of modern medicine he can lead a normal life upon recovery and avoid further heart attacks. If he does everything correctly he could even have a normal life expectancy.

The statistics of heart attacks are appalling. Heart attack has been the leading cause of death in America since 1900. Every 30 seconds an American somewhere suffers a cardiac event. More than half who suffer heart attacks die before ever reaching a hospital. Of those who make it to a hospital to be treated, 60% fail to recover fully.

Everyday I meet patients in my practice. They are diverse as the population in New York where I practice cardiology. Some have mild disease and the others severe. Some disabled by it and others without a symptom. Some are young, others middle aged and some others even in their nineties. They are from different ethnicities and different socio-economic backgrounds. But there is a common denominator among all of them – they all have heart disease-that could have been prevented.

The heart: Art and the science thereof

Heart has been the source of inspiration and imagination to countless artists, poets, dramatists and writers since time immemorial. Heart has been called an organ of fire. Heart is considered the embodiment of courage, audacity, kindness, generosity, love and many other virtues and emotions of nobility and greatness. Heart's romantic impression is as important as its life sustaining vitality in the human being and to that matter in all animals big or small. Heart has been long considered the seat of ones soul where the very essence of life prevailed. This poetic notion is true even in these times of advanced scientific thinking in that incessant and proper functioning of the heart is essential for the sustenance of life. When heart ceases to beat, life itself ceases in that instance.

"Heart is the organ that controls ones life - brain functions only to plan". Above is a valid statement when we consider the vital function of the heart in sustaining life. Heart beats continuously from birth to death. Its rate of function modifies according to the needs of each moment. It beats fast when the body is active or when emotions are stirred. It acts in restful slowness when the body and the mind are at rest. When heart fails to function properly every organ of the body becomes affected. When hearts stops life ends.

The history of the evolution of scientific knowledge of the heart is as interesting as its role in the world of creativity and imagination. The first major landmark discovery in the evolution of modern scientific knowledge of the heart is attributed to the British royal physician Sir William Harvey. In his famous treatise on circulation written in Latin called *De Motu Cordis* Harvey described that blood is circulated around the body and it was the heart that facilitated this circulation. His discovery was the result of painstaking studies he carried out in living animals and human cadavers. He also went onto identify the arteries that carried blood out of the heart to all organs and the far corners of the body and the veins that brought blood back to the heart to be circulated repeatedly around the body in a closed loop fashion.

Since Harvey the science of the heart or cardiology as we call it today had evolved with many more discoveries being made over the years, some epoch making and others not with much fanfare. Development of the stethoscope by the French physician Rene Laennec provided a means by which doctors could examine the heart and its function within the body and make accurate interpretations. The story that led to this discovery too is of some interest. He was faced with the challenge of maintaining decency while listening to a young woman's chest. The usual way of placing ones ear on the bare chest was not the most appropriate of the manners of proper physical examination. So he tried using a hollow tube with one end placed on the patient's chest and the other next to his ear. To his amazement he discovered that not only he could listen to the breathing sounds of the chest but also detailed and amplified sounds made by the various parts of the beating heart. Since then the technology of investigating the heart has advanced to such levels today that doctors can now visualize the beating heart and even the inside cavities of it using ultrasound and other imaging modalities. The stethoscope too has come a long way since the days of Laennec that there are stereophonic stethoscopes that amplify and provide very fine details of heart sounds and computerized digital or "smart" stethoscopes that listen to the heart and make accurate diagnoses and interpretations all by it self.

The other landmark discovery in the evolution of cardiology was the discovery by the Dutch scientist William Einthoven of a means to record the electrical activity of the different areas of the heart from different directions by placing sensors on the body surface. This remarkable discovery earned him the Nobel prize in the early twentieth century. Electrocardiogram thus discovered helps the doctors to identify abnormalities of heart's function by analyzing the changes that happen in the heart's electrical activity. ECG or EKG can provide accurate information about ones heart both of its current status and its history. It is said that the EKG is an accurate record of ones life story. Today doctors can diagnose quite precisely many diseases of the heart simply buy listening to the patient's history, listening to the heart with the stethoscope and analyzing the

EKG. All other cutting-edge technology serves simply to supplement or confirm the inferences thus made.

With the advent of the scientific knowledge, the patterns of the distribution of various diseases of the heart too have evolved. When cardiology and modern medicine was at its infancy in the nineteenth and early twentieth century, most common diseases of the heart were rheumatic heart disease, cardiac syphilis and tuberculosis of the heart. In rheumatic heart disease heart valves are deformed and destroyed by your body's own antibodies that were formed to fight the streptococcus bacteria that caused sore throat. With the advent of antibiotics and better diagnostic and treatment techniques for valve disease theses diseases have become very rare in the contemporary era. Advances made in the areas of public and personal hygiene too have contributed to putting a tab on these communicable diseases. Today the most common heart disease is coronary artery disease.

Advancements in cardiology has shed enormous light into the biggest killer of the contemporary the era, coronary artery disease or ischemic heart disease. This is a disorder of modern day lifestyle of relative physical inactivity and high calorie food intake. Ischemia means inadequate blood supply. The root cause of coronary disease is the gradual narrowing of the coronary arteries compromising the supply of blood to the heart. Most developments in cardiology in the last fifty years have been in the areas of unraveling the mysteries behind the development of ischemic heart disease and its treatment.

The concept and the practicality of inserting wires or narrow tubes called catheters in to the heart via a blood vessel in the groin arm or the neck generated much enthusiasm since its introduction in 1929 by the young German doctor Werner Frossmann. Over the next thirty years this technology progressed rather slowly till 1958 when Mason Sones of the Cleveland clinic started utilizing this modern technology on patients to study the coronary arteries. The arteries thus visualized could be studied for blockages. This led to the development of coronary by pass surgery where surgeons attached veins or arteries taken from elsewhere in the body to bypass the blocked segments of the coronary arteries thus restoring blood flow to the heart. Coronary artery bypass surgery is one of the commonest operations performed worldwide today.

In the nineteen eighties the cardiologists working with catheters demonstrated that hardware such as miniature balloons and other equipment can be introduced to the heart arteries via the catheters to unblock segments of the coronary arteries. This technology developed so rapidly that there is advanced means available today to unblock most coronary arteries thus obviating the necessity for open-heart surgery. However there are limitations to catheter methods where surgery comes to play a major role.

Concept of cardiac catheterization serves not only to unblock coronary arteries. It has shown tremendous use in the areas of investigation and the treatment of electrical abnormalities of the heart. Such abnormalities in the electric circuitry of the heart cause it to beat unusually slowly or extremely rapidly causing symptoms. Doctors introduce electric sensors and transducers via long wires in to the heart to map the electrical activity of the different areas of the heart. If they identify abnormal electric circuits that are causing abnormal rhythms, they burn those with radio frequency energy delivered via a special catheter. This specialized area of cardiology is called cardiac electrophysiology.

In addition catheter technology is used today to close holes in the heart, repair valve abnormalities, replace defective valves and treat other undesirable anatomical abnormalities of the heart.

While the specialty area of interventional cardiology made rapid advances, the specialty area of cardiac imaging utilizing non-invasive means also developed to very high levels of sophistication. The anatomy and the structural details of the beating heart can be studies in great detail by echocardiography where sound beams are used as the means of visualizing the heart. A probe is placed on the surface of the chest, which sends out ultrasound beams that gets reflected back upon hitting the heart. These reflected sound beams are analyzed by a computer that converts the information thus gained into light signals demonstrating the anatomical and functional details of the beating heart. Ultrasound gives vivid details of the heart's pump function, valve function and pressures within the different cavities of the heart.

Radiographic means and magnetic resonance technology (MRI) too have been developed to study the anatomy and the function of the beating heart from outside of the body (by non-invasive means). Use of nuclear isotopes to study the blood supply to the heart and thus diagnose possible coronary artery disease or areas of the heart that has been damaged by heart attacks previously is of significance importance in today's cardiology practice. Nuclear cardiology is the specialized area of cardiology that studies blood supply to the heart this way. This technology involves labeling or tagging blood cells with radioactive atoms and studying the heart for the distribution of this radioactivity using a camera that is sensitive to nuclear radiation. When imaged this way the areas of the heart receiving a good blood supply light up while those areas of the heart not receiving the labeled blood cells remain dark.

In addition to ischemic heart disease or coronary heart disease, heart failure or inability of the heart to pump blood well is also becoming a very prevalent heart disorder in our society. This is more so with the advancement of the average life expectancy and the increased survival of patients after suffering a heart attack. Much attention is focused on the area of research in cardiology to find better means of managing and treating heart failure. In addition to the gradually increasing array of more and more potent drugs in this regard, devices that helps the pump function of the heart called "left ventricle assist devices" (LVADs) are increasingly being used to help millions of patient with severe heart failure.

Everyone is at potential risk of heart disease of some form or the other. The best way to avoid becoming victim to heart disease is not difficult. The most advocated and effective way in this regard is making some simple changes to your lifestyle. The most potent weapon in fighting heart disease is the dissemination of knowledge-making everyone educated on the heart's function and the prevention of its disease. The main objective of this book is to present in an easily understandable and interesting manner the basic facts about your heart and give vital education on how to take control of factors that can harm your heart health. Sound knowledge will help you to protect your heart from potential damage that develop so silently till it raises its ugly head in devastating fury. The old adage "knowledge is power" should be aptly rephrased "knowledge is health and knowledge indeed is life!".

Don's and his dangerous ordeal

"Don how are you feeling?" my question suddenly woke Don up from his short sleep. It took Don another moment to orientate him self to where he was and what was happening around him. Events of the past few hours unfolded in his mind rapidly as he tried to piece together the reality. He could remember going out to mow his lawn in the morning. While at it he started to feel a gradual build up of a tight -pressure like feeling in the middle of his chest. He started to sweat in his face and he felt it becoming increasingly difficult to breath. A terrible sense of anxiety and panic gripped Don as he hurriedly grabbed his cellular phone and dialed "911". Though this has never happened to him before Don knew that something was terribly wrong and that this was the right thing to do. Then he staggered to the nearby garden bench mustering all the energy he could and tried to ease the severe discomfort by resting himself on the bench. But the pain persisted. There was nothing he could do to relieve his chest tightness or the breathlessness. The wait for the ambulance felt like eternity. Don thought he was going to die. Finally the ambulance arrived. The paramedics quickly assessed him, connected him to a cardiac monitor and broke the news "sir it looks like you are having a heart attack…we have to rush you to the nearest hospital". Don heard the paramedic's words, but he had very little insight to comprehend the gravity of the situation. The pain was still too distracting. The paramedic placed an oxygen mask on Don's face while his companion inserted a needle into a vein in his left forearm and started a drip. The paramedics treated Don with a morphine injection through the drip and placed a nitroglycerine tablet under his tongue. Don felt a mild improvement in his terrible discomfort but it still persisted in agonizing severity.

The next moment Don was in the ambulance lying on a stretcher. As they neared the hospital the paramedics received instructions from the doctors to by-pass the emergency room and to transfer Don directly to the cardiac catheterization laboratory. As he was wheeled into the catheterization laboratory I met him for the first time. His pain has eased but he was still quite unwell. I needed to get a clear picture of Don's condition. I questioned him about the details of his current event, his health in the past, his lifestyle and his family health history. Then I did a physical examination and performed an EKG recording of his heart. EKG showed changes consistent with a heart attack in progress. I explained to Don that he was having a massive heart attack and that it was important to treat it in the best possible way immediately. I explained to him that an artery supplying blood to his heart is blocked and the heart muscle in that region will die if the artery is not reopened and blood supply restored. I went on to explain that I could reopen the blocked artery by performing coronary angioplasty. I also described the risks associated with this procedure. But I reassured him that the benefits would far outweigh the potential but rare risks.

Then Don was transferred to the operating table in the catheterization lab and a nurse prepared Don for the procedure. I, upon injecting a local anesthetic agent to Don's right groin accessed his heart arteries with a catheter inserted in to the artery running down to his leg. As I was inserting the needle to his groin I instructed the nurse to give Don a medication to relax. This put Don in to a short slumber. I located the blocked coronary and reopened it. The operation was over within an hour. Don's condition was stable and he had escaped with only very little damage to his heart. He slept through the procedure thanks to the mild sedative I gave him. Don's case was straight forward compared to the case of the young man we discussed before.

Don was still asleep when I saw him in the recovery room half an hour later. Don woke up to my words and turned his head towards me. He was free of the terrible chest tightness and his breathing was back to normal. He felt a tremendous relief. "Don the big artery supplying the bottom wall of your heart was completely blocked off, and that's what was causing your chest pain. You were having a massive heart attack. Luckily the paramedics got to you quickly enough and brought you to us immediately. We unblocked the artery and restored the blood supply to your heart. Any delays could have caused lots of heart muscle damage. This heart attack was severe enough to have even killed you. So it is important that you look after your self very well from here. Your other arteries did not show any significant narrowing" I told Don reassuringly. I left Don promising to him further once he is transferred to the coronary care unit.

Don's story is typical of what happens to millions of Americans every year. There are close to two million admissions to hospital in the US with heart attacks each year. Some having heart attacks that present to a hospital soon enough get prompt treatment that saves valuable heart muscle from permanent damage. Some others sustain considerable damage to their heart before receiving medical help. While there are multitudes of others who fail to reach a hospital alive after a heart attack. That is why knowledge on heart and its health is so important.

Knowledge on heart disease is important to prevent heart disease from developing in those who do not have any heart disease. Those who have heart disease need knowledge on how best to manage them selves so as to minimize chances of further damage or progression of the disease. Those at risk of developing heart disease and those who have heart disease need information on healthy living and on what is in offer out there for their benefit.

Don was lucky in that he did all the right things when he began to experience the symptoms of his heart attack. He made a fast recovery and was discharged from hospital four days later. Before discharge he was commenced on drugs to lower his cholesterol levels and to thin his blood. Don was strongly advised to give up smoking. Don's life changed forever. He had to acquire a great deal of knowledge to change his life style to the better, now that he has been diagnosed with heart disease. He had a positive attitude and he knew by doing the right things he may be able to look forward to a healthier future. Remember, knowledge is health!

Why the Heart Matters

More than 60 million Americans suffer from some form of heart or vascular disease. Heart disease is the biggest killer of all American males above the age of 45 and all American females above the age of 65. It kills more than twice as many people as cancer. One in three males above the age of 60 is considered to be suffering from heart disease. One in ten women aged 45 to 64 has some form of heart disease. This rate increases dramatically to one in five for women over the age of 65 years. In the US close to two million people suffer from heart attacks each year. Approximately one third of the entire adult population in the Western world is considered affected by heart disease in some way. These statistics are considered worse in the highly populated urban areas of the developing countries in Asia and South America. With the improvements made in the areas of prevention and the treatment of heart disease the death rate from coronary heart disease (CHD) has fallen by almost 40 percent over the past 20 years. But in spite of this, the above statistics show that heart disease remains a significant health concern.

The burden of heart disease on the country's healthcare budget is already overwhelming and is projected to become even worse. These costs include health care provision, medication costs as well as costs associated with lost productivity due to the debilitating effects of coronary heart disease. These are staggering numbers for a disease that can be largely prevented by adopting changes to one's lifestyle. Heart disease was largely an unknown disease condition in the latter parts of the 19th century and the early part of the 20th century. Prior to the advent of heart disease into its current epidemic proportions most fatalities among human populations were caused by infectious diseases such the plague, tuberculosis, malaria etc. Most of these diseases have been brought largely under control by the improvements made in sanitation practices, discovery of antibiotics and practice of mass immunization.

Compared to the times before the late nineteenth century majority of the human beings today lead significantly sedentary lives. With the advent of the industrial revolution the energy expenditure of the average human being has gradually and progressively declined. Today it remains at an all time low level. Medical scientists have described an inversely proportionate association between the gradual decrease in physical activity and the increased incidence of coronary heart disease. In addition the calorie and fat content of diet too has gradually increased. Though associated with creature comforts, these changes in human life style has given rise to a number of disease conditions that include coronary heart disease, diabetes, high blood pressure, high cholesterol levels, obesity and stroke. Thus such disorders are called lifestyle disorders. All these unwholesome outcomes of unhealthy lifestyle are interrelated. Often the above disease conditions present together. Therefore knowledge on heart disease should essentially include knowledge on the other diseases mentioned above as well as other risk factors for heart disease. The real value of knowledge is in its ability to make a difference.

The heart and its function

The heart essentially is a pump made of muscle. It beats more than 100,000 times a day. It is located inside the chest cavity behind and towards the left side of the sternum or the breastbone. It weighs approximately 8-14 ounces. There are four cavities within the heart, two on the left and two on the right. The two left sided cavities are separated from the two right-sided cavities by walls made of muscle. The cavities that receive blood into the heart are called atria and the cavities that pump blood out of the heart are called ventricles. Ventricles are more muscular than the thin walled atria. The left ventricle that pumps blood to the whole body except to the lungs is the most muscular cavity of the heart and this is called the main pumping chamber of the heart. The two cavities in the right and the two cavities in left communicate with each other via openings made of valves. These valves direct the blood flow through the heart in a single direction.

Veins are blood vessels (pipes) that enter the right side of the heart bringing blood carrying waste products, especially carbon dioxide, from all over the body. This blood is then pumped to the lungs where carbon dioxide and some other waste material is removed, purified and enriched with oxygen. The oxygen rich blood enters the left side cavities of the heart that pump it to the rest of the body via arteries (muscular pipes). There usually is no communication between the right sided cavities and the left sided cavities of the heart in normal healthy individuals. However there may be minimal communications rarely in some healthy people that would not cause significant health concerns. It has been observed that almost 10% of the population may have a small hole in the septum separating the left atrium from the right atrium. Such small openings are called "patent foramina ovale". Small communications between the left and the right sides are well tolerated by the majority of those who have such defects. But they are at a relatively higher risk of sustaining strokes, migraine headaches and some other symptoms.

A significant communication that causes blood from the right side to mix with that of the left side may lead to ill health. Such communications are popularly known as septal defects. These defects may be found in the septum separating the two arteries or the two ventricles. Most septal defects are congenital and more common among younger individuals. Many such defects gradually close off as one gets old. Septal defects that persist and contribute to health problems may need closing surgically or through interventional means. The latter technique involves placing bio-compatible devices securely occluding the defect by accessing the heart via a blood vessel in the arm or the leg and advancing the device along it.

Heart Muscle

Walls of the four cavities of the heart are made of a specialized muscle structure. This muscle is called "cardiac muscle". Its microscopic structure and function is very similar to the skeletal muscles that are in the arms, legs and elsewhere in the body. But there are few important differences that make cardiac muscle unique and different to skeletal muscle. One major feature of heart muscle is its ability to contract as well regulate contraction by it self. When damaged (as in a heart attack), cardiac muscle has no ability to repair or regenerate. So therefore when damaged cardiac muscle is replaced by scar tissue that has no ability to contribute to the pumping action of the heart.

Heart's electric circuitry

Heart muscle contracts in a synchronized rhythmic manner to facilitate blood flow in a set direction. This synchronized contraction is initiated by an electric signal generator called the cardiac pacemaker. The pacemaker is made up of some very specialized cells and is located in the wall of one of the heart's chambers. These cells generate regular electric signals. The signals generated thus are transmitted all over the heart by a network of special nerve like fibres that act like an electric circuit. Because it conducts electric signals the network made by these fibres is called the cardiac conducting system. Problems in this electric circuitry can lead to disruptions of the normal rhythm of the heart's function. This results in irregular, very rapid or very slow beating of the heart that may bring about symptoms and contribute to other complications. Such disorders of the heart are called rhythm disorders. The specialized area in to the study and the management of such rhythm disorders of the heart is called "cardiac electrophysiology".

Heart Valves

Heart valves are not made of muscle but of a tissue type called fibrous tissue. Valves regulate the blood flow from one cavity in the heart to another and from the heart to the big arteries that carry blood out side. Thus valves ensure forward movement of blood in a single direction. If the valves become leaky or too narrowed it can lead to disease. However diseased valves can be repaired or surgically replaced.

The coronary arteries

The heart muscle requires oxygen and nutrients to pump blood to the lungs and to the rest of the body. It is true that the heart cavities are filled with blood constantly. But it does not supply the heart muscle with blood. The blood vessels that supply the heart muscle with nutrient and oxygen-rich blood are called coronary arteries. These arteries start at the beginning of the aorta, which is the big artery that delivers blood from the main pumping chamber of the heart. Word *corona* means "the crown" in Latin. Since these arteries that supply the heart muscle originate at the top end of the heart like a crown, they are called coronary arteries. These arteries bring oxygen and nutrients to the heart muscle. Two main coronary arteries lie on the surface of the heart. They divide into smaller branches, so that each part of the heart muscle receives oxygen and nutrients. As one gets older these arteries become hard and cholesterol rich material gets deposited in their inner walls. This leads to the narrowing of its inner diameter reducing the amount of blood it can carry. When blood supply to the different parts of the heart is reduced symptoms of angina set in and the ability of the heart to pump blood becomes decreased. This condition is called *atherosclerotic* coronary artery disease and is very common in our society. If a narrowed artery becomes completely blocked, usually by a blood clot, a heart attack takes place. Here the area of the heart muscle to which the blood supply has been abruptly cut off, dies if the artery is not unblocked promptly.

Chapter 2

Coronary artery disease

Proper functioning of the heart is entirely dependent on the constant blood supply to its muscle tissue by the coronary arteries. If the coronary arteries fail to carry enough blood to the heart, its function is compromised. Blood supply to the heart via the coronary arteries can become compromised due to its narrowing by a build up of fatty deposits (plaque) in its walls. Such fatty deposits contain high amounts of cholesterol. These built up of fatty deposits in the inner lining of the coronary arteries become covered with scar tissue gradually clogging up its lumen. This is akin to a metal pipe gradually blocking off due to the build up of rust and other debris in side of it. This process also causes the arteries to harden. This condition is known as plaque disease or *atherosclerosis.* As a result of these blockages, less blood is able to flow through the arteries. Thus the amount of blood that is supplied to the heart muscle is decreased.

Some times blood supply to the heart can become compromised due to the spasm associated narrowing of the coronary arteries. This is a rare situation but is considered equally serious.

How coronary artery disease develops

Deposition of fat and cholesterol in the inner surface of the coronary arteries is considered to start fairly early in your life, particularly if you are at high risk. Over the years such deposits accumulate and their size increases. When the size of such deposits or plaques is big enough to cause significant narrowing of the coronary artery so as to compromise blood supply, the symptoms of angina set in.

Angina

This is the discomfort or the pain you experience when your heart is not getting enough blood supply. Symptoms of angina include a feeling of pressure, tightness or squeezing in the middle of the chest. It may also cause aching behind the breastbone. Some may experience a feeling similar to that of heartburn or stomach-ache. Angina can also take the form of cramping in the chest or pain that spreads to the arms, neck, jaws or back of the chest. This may also accompany a feeling of fatigue or shortness of breath.

Exertional or Stable angina

This is angina experienced on physical exertion. When muscles of the body become active there is a need for its blood supply to be increased by several folds. This places an increased demand on the heart to increase its pump function by contracting harder and faster. In healthy individuals with healthy coronary arteries blood supply to the working heart can increase by several folds to meet the increased demand for oxygen and nutrients. If there is narrowing in the coronary arteries the blood supply cannot be augmented as required. This leads to a lack of oxygen to the working heart muscle and the accumulation of waste products in the affected area leading to the development of angina pain. This symptom is called exertional angina because it is triggered by physical exertion. Effort related angina is very suggestive of the presence of significant narrowing (more that 60% of the internal diameter) of the coronary arteries. This development however does not warn of an imminent heart attack. Therefore angina associated with exertion is also called "stable angina". Exertional or stable angina warrants further investigation and treatment by a cardiologist expeditiously.

Unstable angina

Significant and sudden narrowing of coronary arteries can lead to the development of angina while at rest. This situation usually is very suggestive of an imminent heart attack thus needs to be managed at a hospital emergency department. Angina that develops at rest is called unstable angina.

Heart attack/Myocardial infarction

If sudden worsening of the narrowing of a coronary artery leads to completed blockade of the artery it will cut off blood supply to the relevant area of the heart muscle. This is called a myocardial infarction or a heart attack. Heart muscle is unable to survive for more than a few minutes without blood supply, and therefore during a heart attack the affected area of the heart is damaged and the affected heart muscle dies. Heart attack causes prolonged and continuous angina like chest discomfort in a much severe manner. In addition there can be increased sweating with the feeling of nausea and vomiting. Some may experience sudden onset shortness of breath or light-headedness. But in contrast some others, particularly those who suffer from diabetes, may not experience any chest discomfort associated with heart attack at all. Thus the heart attack may go unnoticed. This is called a "silent infarction". Heart attack or myocardial infarction is a life threatening medical emergency and needs to be managed in a hospital emergency room urgently. There is treatment to unblock an occluded coronary artery to restore blood supply to the affected area of the heart. Restoration of blood supply to the affected area of the heart should be done urgently. The earlier the blood supply is restored the more heart muscle can be salvaged form damage. This damage or threatened damage to the heart is what happens in a heart attack.

Who is at risk?

Coronary heart disease is very common in our society. Everyone is potentially at risk of developing this condition. However some are at a higher risk than others. Certain factors are known to increase ones risk of developing atherosclerosis or blockages in the coronary arteries. These factors are defined as "risk factors` for coronary artery disease. Following is a list of recognized such risk factors-

* Aging
* Diabetes mellitus
* Heredity or genetics (family history)
* High blood pressure
* High cholesterol levels
* Obesity
* Smoking
* Male gender
* Physical inactivity
* Race

Many of the above factors can be changed and brought under control by changing your life style or by taking medications. Such changeable or controllable risk factors are called "modifiable coronary risk factors". The risk factors that cannot be controlled include age, gender, race and heredity.

The more risk factors you have the higher the risk of developing heart disease becomes. Thus the risk factors have an additive effect. A person suffering from high blood pressure and diabetes who continues to smoke cigarettes may have a 10 to 20 times higher risk of developing heart disease than an individual without any risk factors.

Can coronary heart disease be prevented?

Presence of risk factors does not mean that you have already developed heart disease. Identification and addressing of risk factors can prevent heart disease in those who have not developed it as yet. The risk factors such as age, gender, race and family history cannot be changed. Earlier you are able to identify your risk factors and take appropriate measures to control or minimize their impact the better are the chances of preventing coronary heart disease from developing. The first step to controlling risk factors is to educate your self in this regards.

Age

Your risk of developing heart disease increases with advancing age. However, the onset of atherosclerosis is known to start fairly early in life. In the post mortem studies carried out in the young soldiers that were killed in combat during the Korean war doctors found evidence of early stages of coronary artery disease in the coronary arteries. But what is even more startling is the discovery of early evidence of cholesterol deposition in the coronary arteries of the still borne fetuses of high-risk parents. Thus the development of coronary artery disease is described as a process that starts very early in life and progress over a long period of time. But the important fact to remember is that you would not know that you have got coronary heart disease till it has developed to a fairly advanced stage so as to block the artery to a significant degree. This usually happens as you approach middle age or later. Majority of the males get diagnosed with coronary heart disease in the mid to late sixties. For females it is the early to mid seventies. But patients are known to present as early as in their twenties, however this is very rare. Those that present with significant coronary artery disease before the age of thirty usually (but not invariably) have an inherited disease condition that causes the rapid development and progression of coronary artery disease. Some disorders of cholesterol metabolism and a disease called homocystinurea are some such conditions that cause heart attacks at a very young age. Abuse of narcotics such as cocaine too can cause the development of heart disease at an early age. Doctors can estimate your risk of developing heart disease fairly early by studying your cardiac risk factors.

Gender

Males are at a higher risk of developing heart disease. But however after menopause the risk of females developing heart disease gradually increases to become equal to that of the males by the age of about sixty-five years. The increased susceptibility of the male patient to coronary heart disease is partly attributed to the male hormone testosterone. There has been evidence to suggest that there is rapid progression of coronary heart disease in some individuals who receive testosterone as a therapy for other medical conditions.

The relative protection from coronary heart disease the females enjoy is attributed to the female sex hormone estrogen. The precise mechanism by which estrogen exercises this protection is still not conclusively described. It is well known that estrogen has beneficial effects on controlling blood cholesterol levels.

For a while there was a belief in the medical community that replacing the hormone estrogen in women after menopause would help protect them from developing heart disease. But the latest research carried out to ascertain the validity of the above hypothesis has shown that replacement of estrogen (hormone replacement therapy) in fact can increase your chances of developing heart disease after menopause. It is obvious that estrogen behaves in opposite ways in the pre menopausal and post-menopausal women. A logical explanation to this phenomenon is still awaited.

Family History

Family history of a first-degree relative developing heart disease increases your predisposition to developing heart disease. This is more so if the first-degree relative had developed coronary heart disease before the age of 60. This is an inherited risk and suggests a genetic association in the development of heart disease. It is believed that coronary heart disease is associated with many different genes. Therefore it is called a "multigenic" disorder.

Cardiovascular genetics and the inherited nature of coronary heart disease still remain largely unexplained. However researches have already identified several genes that if present, can increase your risk of developing coronary heart disease. This is an area of medical research that is gaining momentum very fast. One can expect many exciting and interesting developments to take place in this area in the time to come.

Race

There is a racial bias to the risk of developing heart disease. African Americans, Indigenous Americans, Australian aborigines and South Asian ethnics have a relatively higher tendency to develop coronary artery disease compared to the Caucasians and the East Asians. They also tend to develop heart disease much earlier in life. In these individuals coronary artery disease more often present in a much severe form. This racial bias once again is attributed to an interplay of genetics and environment.

It is interesting to know that this increased risk of developing coronary heart disease in the above mentioned races is high only among those oriented to a western life style. So the increased prevalence of heart disease is seen in those living in urban areas of their countries of origin or those who have migrated to the West. Presence of coronary heart disease is very minimal and at times almost non-existent among those living in the rural and traditional settings. Researchers have explained this trend as being due to the genes that are switched on or activated by the change to the western way of living. This is another instance where genetic factors and environmental factors interact with each other to cause the development of a disease.

Smoking

Cigarette smoking is a very strong risk factor for coronary heart disease. Higher the number of cigarettes you smoke the higher the risk. However, even one cigarette a day is considered a significant risk. The exact mechanism by which cigarette smoking causes heart disease is still not clearly explained. The chemical constituent of cigarette smoke that mediates this risk too has not been defined yet. But observational and epidemiological studies have established a direct and definite risk associated with smoking.

Smoking of tobacco by other means such as cigars and pipes too can increase the risk of heart disease but to a lesser degree than with cigarettes. In addition to causing disease in the coronary arteries, smoking can cause disease in the arteries elsewhere in the body too. Smoking is a direct risk factor for peripheral arterial disease where one develops narrowing of the arteries supplying blood to the legs and feet. Patients suffering from this condition experience leg pain on walking. In much severe forms it progresses to non-healing or poorly healing ulcers in the feet and even to the death of toes. By contributing to the narrowing of the arteries supplying blood to the brain, cigarette smoking acts as a risk factor for stroke.

Those who are treated for coronary artery disease by coronary artery by pass surgery or balloon angioplasty and stenting develop rapid narrowing of the bypass grafts or the stents that are placed in the arteries if they continue to smoke. The mortality rates of those who continue to smoke after such a procedure is several folds higher than those who do not. It is said that women have a higher risk of heart disease associated with smoking than men.

Obesity

Obesity is another modifiable risk factor for heart disease. Obesity is usually the net effect of excess calorie intake and relative physical inactivity. In addition to heart disease, obesity can increase the risk of stroke, certain cancers, diabetes and high blood pressure. Due to its ability to cause disease, obesity increases your mortality. The best way to define obesity is by calculating the body mass index. Body mass index is calculated by dividing your body weight measured in kilograms by the squared value of your height in meters. A body mass index of less than 25 is considered ideal. Between 25 and 29.9 is defined as over weight and any value above 30 is considered obese.

The pattern of distribution of body fat too has an important role to play in your predisposition to heart disease. Central obesity where body fat is predominantly distributed in the abdominal region is considered more risky than fat deposition elsewhere. This type of obesity is more common among males and is called android obesity. This is also associated with a higher risk of high blood pressure, cholesterol elevation and diabetes.

Diabetes

Diabetes is a modifiable risk factor for coronary heart disease. Diabetes causes disease in the coronary arteries as well as other small and larger arteries in the body. In addition to coronary heart disease, diabetes is a risk factor for stroke and kidney disease. Diabetes associated risk for heart disease is so significant that those with diabetes are advised to be treated as having had a heart attack already. In addition to controlling blood sugar levels adequately, diabetics should also be treated with other heart protecting medications given to the patients who have been already diagnosed with heart disease. Diabetics usually tend to have very diffuse disease in the coronary arteries.

High blood pressure

Long standing blood pressure is a significant risk factor for heart disease. High blood pressure causes coronary arteries as well arteries elsewhere in the body to become stiff and diseased. Just like diabetes, high blood pressure too is a cause for stroke as well as kidney disease. Good control of blood pressure is a must in the prevention and the treatment of heart disease. High blood pressure is also the leading cause of heart failure world-wide. High blood pressure can be caused by many factors. However over 95% patients suffering from high blood pressure have no causative factor behind their disease condition. This is called essential high blood pressure or essential hypertension.

High cholesterol levels

Cholesterol is a major component of the atherosclerotic plaque that builds up in the inner lining of the coronary artery that causes its narrowing. There are different types of cholesterol in the blood. Most of the cholesterol found in the blood is manufactured in the liver. The other major source of cholesterol is food. Recommended safe cholesterol level of each individual depends on the absence or the presence of other coronary risk factors. The three main types of cholesterol of interest are LDL, HDL and triglycerides. Of these it is desirable to have LDL and triglycerides as low as possible and HDL as high as possible.

Cholesterol levels can be controlled to a certain degree by dieting and regular physical exercise. If these measures fail to bring the blood cholesterol level under control drugs can be prescribed. There are drugs with high potency to control cholesterol very effectively.

Physical inactivity

Relative physical inactivity is considered a fundamental cause behind heart disease and other lifestyle disorders. Physical inactivity causes excess energy consumed as food to be stored as fat. Thus it causes weight gain. Physical inactivity also causes your heart to lose efficiency and conditioning. In contrast physical activity has been shown to be effective in reducing the incidence of heart disease as well as deaths from heart disease. Other beneficial effects of regular physical activity include lowering of blood pressure, controlling of blood sugar levels, improvement in blood cholesterol level and weight loss.

Socio-economics

Scientists and doctors that study the distribution of diseases in different population groups have discovered that there is a definite difference in the prevalence of coronary heart disease in populations belonging to the different social classes divided on the average income and the level of education. Coronary heart disease is much more common among those earning lower incomes and employed in blue collar or manual/unskilled vocations. In addition such populations had a higher distribution of all coronary risk factors including high blood pressure, diabetes, smoking, high cholesterol levels and obesity. Risk of heart disease was high among those who were relatively ignorant on issues of health and good health related practices.

How can you reduce your risk?

Even though heart disease usually develops after middle age the onset of the process of plaque build up in the arteries and atherosclerosis happens much earlier in your life. So the process of controlling your risk factors too should start as early as possible. First step towards risk factor modification is to acquire good knowledge about your personal risk and risk factors. Your doctor can help you calculate your absolute risk of developing heart disease within the next ten years.

High blood pressure, high blood cholesterol levels, high blood glucose levels in diabetes and obesity can be brought under control first by increasing your leisure time physical activity, physical exercise and by planning and controlling your diet. If such non-medical means fail to control blood pressure, blood cholesterol levels, blood sugar levels and cause weight reduction, appropriate medications should be commenced. Smoking has to be stopped and if you find it hard to give up smoking you can be helped with counseling and medications.

Addressing risk factors involve changing your life style, diet, habits and may be perhaps taking tablets to control the risk factors that would not come under satisfactory control by lifestyle changes alone. First it is important to know your risk factors. Once known it is important to check whether they are under control. Once under control the risk factors should be monitored constantly to ensure that their control is maintained. Basic steps in risk factor control are as follows-

- Control blood pressure if high
- Stop smoking
- Lose weight if over weight (if your weight is more than what is appropriate for your height)
- Control blood sugar levels if diabetic
- Control cholesterol levels if high
- Relax and de-stress
- Commence physical exercise
- Get your self checked up with your doctor regularly

As with anything in life it easier said than done. But if you are motivated enough there is nothing that is too difficult to do to change in the way you live. Knowing that you need to change to save your own life is the beginning of the process. I intend to give you that knowledge that is necessary to make a fresh start in your life. Once you know that you have to change, it is important to know how you can change. In addition I intend to educate you on the help that is available widely to make the process of change possible. Controlling the above-mentioned traditional coronary risk factors is the basic step to healthy living. In addition incorporating some wonderful additions to your life style in the way of healthy practices and habits may further enhance the quality of your life. I will be discussing all this in the light of modern scientific thinking in the chapters to come.

Chapter 3

The cholesterol factor

The plaque deposits that cause the blockages in the coronary arteries are rich in cholesterol. Similar plaques can deposit in the inner walls of many other arteries in the body and cause blockages. High blood cholesterol levels have been identified as a direct risk factor responsible for promoting such cholesterol deposits. Therefore it is absolutely necessary that blood cholesterol level be kept under adequate control. There has been a great amount of research work carried out looking into the significance of cholesterol level and the means of cholesterol reduction. Tremendous progress has been made in uncovering the ways by which high cholesterol levels cause problems and how best to control its impact. The amount of knowledge uncovered in this area of interest in cardiology is truly amazing. A specialized area of medical sciences has evolved called “lipidology” that specifically studies lipids and in particular cholesterol. The knowledge on cholesterol is growing even more rapidly as more and more research work is being carried out. In addition this research has led to the development of an array of drugs that seem to do wonders in protecting those who are at risk of developing heart disease and those who have heart disease. Furthermore these agents seem to provide promise in other areas of medicine too.

What is cholesterol?

Cholesterol is a chemical substance similar to fat. Cholesterol can be produced out of fat substances. Cholesterol is necessary for body’s normal function. Body in fact can fulfill all of its cholesterol needs by producing it within the body itself. Many hormones in the body are derived of cholesterol. In addition we ingest cholesterol with our food. Animal fats have cholesterol in high amounts. Egg yolk is a very rich source of cholesterol. In addition saturated fats in the food we eat promote the formation cholesterol in increased amounts in our body.

Though cholesterol in right amounts is necessary for body's healthy function, presence of it in the blood in excess amounts can lead to deleterious health effects. The main health complication of high blood cholesterol levels is the plaque formation in the inner wall of arteries. Narrowing and blockage of arteries due to these plaques cause coronary heart disease, stroke, kidney disease and many other problems of poor circulation and disrupted organ function.

Types of cholesterol

There are many different types of cholesterol in our body and some are considered very bad while others are considered beneficial or good. When checking cholesterol levels doctors usually measure the levels of three main types of cholesterol. In addition the total cholesterol level too is recorded.

LDL cholesterol or low-density lipoprotein cholesterol is one of the bad forms of cholesterol. This type of cholesterol causes and promotes the plaque deposition in the inner walls of arteries. Higher the level of LDL higher the risk of developing heart disease. HDL cholesterol or high-density lipoprotein cholesterol on the other hand is the good type of cholesterol. It has the ability to prevent the build up of cholesterol in the blood stream and prevent plaque deposition in the arteries. Third type of cholesterol is called triglycerides and is another bad form. This too contributes to increase the risk of heart disease. It can also cause inflammation and disease of the pancreas. It is desirable to lower the levels of LDL cholesterol and triglycerides and increase the levels of HDL cholesterol.

High Cholesterol levels

There are many factors that would cause the blood cholesterol levels to go up. Intake of rich fatty food, obesity and physical inactivity are the commonest causes for this condition. Genetic factors too play a major role in determining cholesterol levels in the blood. There are genetic disorders that cause huge elevations of blood cholesterol levels even in young individuals leading to early and at times fatal heart disease. Due to lifestyle factors any adult in our society is at high risk of developing high blood cholesterol levels. Elevated cholesterol levels it self does not cause symptoms therefore many may not realize that they are at high risk of developing heart disease due to high cholesterol levels. So therefore it cannot be overemphasized the importance of checking your blood cholesterol levels if you are over 35 years of age or have other risk factors for heart disease. Once diagnosed and treated it is advisable to check cholesterol levels every six months to ensure good control.

Desirable cholesterol levels

Blood cholesterol levels can go up transiently after a meal. Due to this reason, to get an accurate reading, blood cholesterol has to be checked after an over night fast (at least 11 hours). Recommended or desirable blood cholesterol levels have been decreased gradually over the last few years promoting tighter and tighter control. This is due to each new drug trial investigating the benefits of cholesterol control showing better benefits from further reduction in the cholesterol levels-far below the recommended levels of the time. Therefore today's guidelines may soon change to recommend even tighter control in the future. However the bottom line of this fact is that the lower the total cholesterol, LDL cholesterol and triglyceride levels are the better and more beneficial it is for your health. In a similar manner higher the HDL level the better it is for good cardiac health. Current recommendation for ideal cholesterol level depends on your level of risk for developing heart disease.

Total cholesterol level

In general total cholesterol level is ideal to be maintained below 200 mg/dL. Any level above 240 mg/dL is considered high and warranting treatment.

LDL cholesterol level

A LDL cholesterol level below 100 mg/dL is considered ideal. Any level above 160mg/dL is considered high warranting treatment. Based on the evidence from the latest trials on cholesterol lowering therapy doctors increasingly recommend very low LDL cholesterol levels as being more beneficial. The current recommendation is therefore to bring down the LDL cholesterol levels below 70 mg/dL. The trials showed that lower the LDL levels more the benefits are.

HDL cholesterol

HDL cholesterol should be maintained above the level of 45 mg/dL in males and above 55 mg/dL in females. HDL levels above 60mg/dL render good protection from heart disease. With the evidence from the cholesterol lowering trials many doctors have begun to identify the unique and important role of HDL in promoting heart health. The next focus on cholesterol management is possibly going to solely on the ways of elevating the levels of this good cholesterol variety. This is such an important fact that some doctors have correctly summarized that all cholesterol types that is not an HDL is bad and should be suppressed. Scientific evidence in fact suggest that elevating HDL not only prevents future build up of cholesterol deposits in the blood vessels but also decreases thickness of the plaques that have been deposited in the past, perhaps may be over a life time.

Some times statin drugs alone may not bring about sufficient elevation of HDL levels in some patients. In such situations “Niacin” too should be added to complement the activity of statins.

Triglyceride levels

Triglyceride levels should be maintained below 150mg/dL. A level above 200 mg/dL is dangerous and need drug treatment.

Guidelines for the treatment of high cholesterol levels

Currently the general guidelines are aimed at primarily controlling LDL cholesterol level.

If you have diabetes or heart disease: In any individual who has been diagnosed with coronary heart disease or has diabetes, the LDL cholesterol level should be ideally maintained at a level below 100 mg/dL. If the levels are between 100 and 129 mg/dL, therapeutic life style changes should be initiated with the aim of bringing the cholesterol level to or below 100 mg/dL. If the LDL cholesterol level is above 130 mg/dL, cholesterol lowering drug therapy should be considered.

If you have risk factors only: In individuals having two or more coronary risk factors (high blood pressure, positive family history of heart disease, male above 45 or female above 55 or post menopausal, cigarette smoking or HDL cholesterol level below 40mg/dL) the LDL cholesterol level should be maintained below 130 mg/dL. If it is above this value therapeutic life style changes should be initiated. Any value above 160 mg/dL warrants drug therapy.

If you are risk free at minimal risk : In individuals at minimal risk (with nil or one coronary risk factor) LDL cholesterol level should be maintained below 160 mg/dL. Levels between 160-190 mg/dL warrants initiation of therapeutic lifestyle changes. Any level above 190mg/dL necessitates treatment with drugs.

(NCEP Expert panel. Executive summary of the Third Report of the National Cholesterol Education Program (NCEP) Expert Panel on Detection, Evaluation, and treatment of High Blood Cholesterol in Adults (Adult Treatment Panel III). Bethesda, MD: National Heart, Lung and Blood Institute, National Institute of

Health; 2001. NIH publication 01-3670).

How to manage cholesterol levels

Management of high blood cholesterol level starts with the initiation of therapeutic or healthy lifestyle changes unless the levels are extremely high. Research has convincingly shown that initiation and maintenance of therapeutic life style changes can bring about significant improvements (almost up to 10% reduction) in the blood cholesterol levels. Consumption of food with low on no fat and low calories is an integral dietary change. In addition food with mono unsaturated fatty acids, fresh fruits, high-fiber foods and green vegetables should be consumed more. Those food products that contain plant stanols or plant sterols (for example, cholesterol-lowering margarines) have good cholesterol lowering capabilities. Soya products too have been found out to be very beneficial in this regard. Regular physical exercise should be commenced and carried out continuously. This may take the form of moderate intensity exercise for at least for 30 minutes performed four times a week. Weight loss should be another goal of importance. In addition other coronary risk factors if present should be addressed accordingly.

Where above life style changes fail to achieve anticipated cholesterol goals, drug treatment has to be initiated.

Cholesterol lowering drugs

Many types of cholesterol lowering drugs have evolved very rapidly over the last ten years. Today, as a result of intense research and medical trials, there are many very powerful cholesterol lowering drugs available to those needing treatment. Their side effects and tolerability too have significantly improved compared to the earlier agents. Statin drugs comprise the mainstay of cholesterol treatment today. Statins have shown remarkable benefits in decreasing the incidence of heart attacks and reducing mortality among the participants in many large trials. The commonly prescribed "statin"

drugs (simvastatin -zocor, artovastatin - lipitor, pravastatin – pravachol) are capable of lowering both types of bad cholesterol, LDL and triglycerides. Where necessary other traditional agents used in the past can be added on to the statin agent to get a better control of your cholesterol profile. These other drugs used for treating high cholesterol levels include bile acid sequestrants (cholestyramine), gemfibrozil, probucol and nicotinic acid (niacin). These drugs are used less frequently now. However nicotinic acid and gemfibrozil help in the control of very high triglyceride levels.
Fish oil too has a potent ability to control blood cholesterol levels. A well-publicized study called GISSI (an Italian acronym) by an Italian group demonstrated that fish oil consumption could decrease mortality due to cardiovascular disease.

"Lp little a"

Lp(a) or "*lipoprotein little a*" is another type of cholesterol that has been implicated as a causative factor for atherosclerotic heart disease. Elevated levels of Lp(a) is said to be a main contributor to the development of heart disease in those with normal levels of conventional cholesterol sub types. There is much research work being carried out currently to identify exactly how Lp(a) acts in the development of heart disease and the means of best controlling it. Nicotinic acid has been identified as the best agent to control the elevated levels of Lp(a). Nicotinic acid doses that could reduce Lp(a) levels by 10-25% was shown to decrease mortality rates due to heart disease among the participants in a trial called the CDP or the Coronary Drug Project trial. Doctors do not routinely check Lp(a) levels. Discuss with your doctor whether it is important to check and treat if necessary, your Lp(a) level.

Estrogen and cholesterol

The female sex hormone estrogen too has potent cholesterol lowering effects. It is known to decrease the levels of LDL as well as Lp(a) while increasing the levels of the good cholesterol HDL.

The only catch with estrogen is its effect of elevating the bad form of cholesterol triglycerides. Doctors who studied the benefits of estrogen in controlling heart disease showed that estrogen while improving cholesterol levels failed to reduce the incidence of heart disease. These facts came to light in the study called HERS or Heart and Estrogen Replacement Study.

The evolution of statin drugs

The rise and evolution of statin drugs essentially changed the practice of cardiology in the contemporary era. It is a major factor that also changed the face of modern medicine. Statin drugs block a key enzyme that helps produce cholesterol in the body. Since its discovery researchers have carried out many clinical trial to ascertain the efficacy and the usefulness of this drug. As per common practice these trial have been given catchy names, which are acronyms of the descriptive titles of the studies.

The life saving benefits of statin drugs in the primary prevention of coronary heart disease (in those who were at risk of heart disease but did not have a diagnosis of the same) was first shown in two large clinical trials called the WOSCOPS study and the AFCAPS/TexCAPS study. WOSCOPS stands for West of Scotland Coronary prevention Study and AFCAPS/TexCAPS stands for Air Force/Texas Coronary Atherosclerosis Prevention Study.
Studies that showed the life saving benefits of statin drugs in those who have had heart attacks (secondary prevention) are the 4S study, LIPID study, CARE study and HPS study. They showed that stain drugs reduced the incidence of heart attacks and death due to heart disease in those who were treated. 4S stands for Scandinavian Simvastatin Survival Study, LIPID stands for Long-term Intervention with Pravastatin in Ischemic Disease, CARE stands for Cholesterol and Recurrent Events Trial and HPS for Heart Protection Study.
These landmark studies established the absolute benefits of treatment with statin drugs. Due to the results of these studies statins have become some of the most commonly prescribed drugs

all over the world.

Overall satins could decrease LDL levels by 25%-40% and triglyceride levels by 10%-30%. In a similar manner statins decreased the relative risk of major adverse cardiac events (heart attack, stroke or death) by 25-40%. These studies showed that regular treatment with statin drugs reduced the incidence of fatal and non fatal heart attacks and also death due to other heart conditions. These landmark trial not only established the potent efficacy of statin drugs in controlling blood cholesterol levels but also proved the value of these agents in preventing all major cardiovascular events (death, heart attack, stroke) and saving lives.

Another remarkable discovery was made in two of the statin studies (Heart Protection Study and ASCOT - Anglo Scandinavian Cardiac Outcomes Trial). According to the results of these studies, even those with normal cholesterol levels when treated with statin drugs, reap health benefits just as those with a high cholesterol levels.

Another consequence of these trials was the progressive lowering of the recommended blood cholesterol level for the prevention of cardiovascular disease. At one instance some healthcare workers got so excited about the beneficial effects of statins that they suggested that it be added to public drinking water supplies!

Though there is convincing evidence to the life saving value of statin drugs to those with coronary heart disease and those at risk of developing coronary artery disease, many of those who should be on it do not seem to be taking it due to numerous reasons. When started early after a heart attack, statins can decrease the mortality of the patient by a significant level. However researchers have revealed that only 40% of those with high cholesterol actually get started on statin therapy after a heart attack. In addition other surveys have revealed that 40% of those on stating therapy for high cholesterol levels do not get high enough of a dose to control cholesterol levels adequately. So there is a definite need for the review of statin prescription patterns for those with or at risk of heart disease. This should include better education of the prescribing doctors as well as the patients or those individuals at risk.

Main side effects of concern with the use of statin drugs were inflammation or pain in the muscles, liver abnormalities and rare allergies. The large clinical trials proved that these side effects are extremely rare and failed to compromise the hugely beneficial effects of taking the drug.

Other benefits of statin drugs

Statin agents are known to confer more health benefits than simply bringing down blood cholesterol levels and prevent heart disease. Statins are known to act as anti-inflammatory agents. They have also been observed to be able to prevent Alzheimer's disease of old age. Researchers have observed that statins could reduce the degeneration of pig valves in those who have had heart valve replacement. The greatest shortcoming of pig valves used in the treatment of valve disease is its degeneration over time leading to recurrent valve malfunctioning and heart failure.

The Italian connection

There is a tremendous amount of scientific work being carried out to find new and better forms of cholesterol lowering therapies. One such cutting edge treatment being developed started with scientists in 1974 observing that the people in a tiny Italian village called Limone sul Garda just outside of Milan living long lives without developing heart disease. The most interesting observation was that despite their longevity they had very high levels of bad cholesterol LDL and very low levels of good cholesterol HDL. After studying these people for a while scientists discovered that they had a mutant form of a protein called apolipoprotein-A1 that prevented cholesterol plaques forming in their arteries. The scientists named this protein "apolipoprotein-A1 Milano". Scientists then went on to show that injecting artificially synthesized apo-A1 Milano could in fact prevent coronary artery disease in high-risk individuals.

Recently a small pilot study that injected artificially synthesized HDL or good cholesterol into those with heart disease and high cholesterol levels showed that it could clear the blocked arteries. More research is being carried out in this regard. This break through promises exciting new therapies to fight cholesterol and heart disease in the future.

Cholesterol management has become a focal point in the quest to beat heart disease. While more and more new drugs to fight cholesterol are being developed the sole onus for your cholesterol management still remains to be on you. Life style changes with the control of diet and increased physical activity and strict compliance with medications will ensure good cholesterol control in you. This may reward you with a healthy life and a long life.

Chapter 4

Lose weight-Gain health and happiness

Martha is 50 years old. I have known her for almost six months now. She was referred to me by an endocrinologist colleague who was concerned about the shortness of breath that she was experiencing even on minimal exertion. He suspected Martha to have coronary artery disease and perhaps heart failure. She was obese and diabetic. Her body weight was 310 pounds and her body mass index as I calculated was 34. I liked Martha as a patient. She was intelligent and had a good insight into her medial condition. She knew that her obesity was a challenge she had to overcome. She has always been in the larger side of the divide. But she had gained most her excess weight after her last pregnancy 22 years ago. She had tried occasionally dieting but without an evident success. She developed diabetes at the age of 40. She also had high blood pressure and her cholesterol levels were higher than the normal limits. She was largely sedentary. Her attempts at doing some physical exercise did not go beyond just planning. Lack of motivation and painful arthritis in her knees were other factors that prevented Martha from exercising.

She smoked about 20 cigarettes a day. This was her coping mechanism for the mental stress she experienced with her eating habits. She knew that she was over eating. She had such an unsatiable appetite that she had to eat some thing practically every half-hour. Her repertoire of "snacks" included chocolates, potato chips, pastries, cakes and many other forms of fast food. She could not control her cravings however much she tried. It was a real battle. Not eating when she felt hungry made her distressed. This made her smoke cigarettes. Then she felt little relaxed. This relaxed feeling gave her a false sense of confidence that it is okay to eat. Then she ate to satisfy her craving. After eating she felt guilty and remorseful. The mental distress associated with this feeling of remorse made her smoke. So this situation kept repeating like a cycle. As a result she was gaining more and more weight. In the background she constantly felt depressed and dejected.

At our first meeting we discussed mostly her symptoms of breathlessness. She was short of breath even while at rest at times. She could not lie down for more than half an hour because she developed breathing difficulty. She never experienced chest pain. But again because Martha is diabetic she could have coronary artery disease and even heart attacks without ever experiencing chest pain. Martha had a bad combination of cardiac risk factors in the form of her obesity, high blood pressure, diabetes and high cholesterol levels. And to top it all she smoked cigarettes fairly heavily. Martha sure was sitting on a time bomb. A heart attack could strike any moment with deadly and devastating consequences.

I discussed the seriousness of her symptoms and organized her admission to hospital for investigations and treatment. I believed her breathlessness was due to multiple factors. But all these factors were directly linked to her obesity. My urgent concern was the shape of her heart and the coronary arteries. Heart trouble would be the one that would take her life first! I performed a coronary angiogram on her the very next day and my suspicion was correct. (Prior to getting Martha on the table I had to check with the manufacturer whether the operating table could handle Martha's weight). Martha had multiple narrowings in two of her three main coronary arteries. I decided to open the blocked arteries with angioplasty and place the new drug-coated stents to prevent them from re narrowing. The intervention was challenging. Her arteries were small and badly diseased. Martha's heart was very sensitive that even a short period of reduced blood supply to heart muscle was not tolerated. Her obesity made her body anatomy more difficult to work through. With meticulous manipulation I opened all the blocked arteries one by one and the placed the stents.

The operation though risky, arduous and prolonged, was a success. But all was not well – Martha had a challenging uphill task ahead of her to change her life style to prevent recurrence of coronary disease and avoid early death. If she were to continue her life style I assured her that her arteries would re narrow in no time. And there was a real possibility that she would not make it to a hospital alive the next time. If a stent in her coronary arteries were to block off suddenly due to a clot cutting off blood supply to a large area of her heart, she would die in an instant. Smoking is one big risk factor for clot formation in stents shortly after intervention.

I had a long discussion with her the same evening in the recovery room of the catheterization laboratory. In the course of our conversation Martha wept. She felt desperately helpless. She believed that she was a victim of her own lack of will and resolve. She pleaded me for help to give up smoking and lose weight. I told her that the best and the most effective way to stop smoking is to give up completely and straight away or in other words "go cold turkey". She said she was ready for that despite the cravings she was fighting after a whole day without a cigarette. I prescribed nicotine patches to ease her cravings – which are both psychological as well as neurological manifestations of nicotine dependence. I also organized the cardiac nutritionist to see her before her discharge the next day to formulate a dietary plan to lose weight. In addition I commenced her on blood thinning tablets, a blood pressure medication and a statin drug to lower cholesterol.

The next morning I saw Martha again before her discharge. I was very concerned about her. She had a tremendous task to make an absolute U-turn in her life style. I was particularly concerned about her psychological state. Martha's mind was the key to facilitating change herself. So my strategy was first to impart a sense of urgency and cultivate in her mind as much motivation as possible. As the first step I gave Martha some pep talk and encouraged her to look at the great rewards of taking control of her lifestyle and losing weight. All these rewards- better health, physical attractiveness, social appeal, better image, zest and vitality were highly attractive to her. Then I referred her to a psychologist colleague for further galvanize her will power and motivation. On consultation with a nutritionist I formulated a dietary plan for her. This plan involved diets predominantly made up of fresh vegetable, fresh fruits, nuts, legumes and fiber. She also learned about the different calorie values of her food and how to count the calories of her meals. Thus she developed the practice of controlling her daily calorie intake. I strongly recommended regular physical exercise as much as she could tolerate and also referred her to a yoga instructor known to me. Over time I observed Martha's thought processes changing. She was becoming more and more assertive and in control of her lifestyle. This health conscious mentality made her to comply well with the plans we drew up together for her weight loss. She stuck to her diet, exercised regularly and continued attending yoga classes. In a year she lost over hundred and fifty pounds. With weight loss blood pressure came back to normal levels, her blood sugar levels became normal and so did her cholesterol levels. I could stop her blood pressure pills and diabetes tablets altogether. The painful arthritis of her knees disappeared. She has not had any recurrence of her heart disease over the year that I have been looking her after.

Obesity - a modern epidemic

Martha's was an unusual success story. But the majority who experience similar circumstances fails to do so well. Each year, obesity causes almost half a million excess deaths. Obesity is a major health problem in the western world. But it is also increasingly becoming prevalent in the developing countries. It is identified as a health problem that is growing in epidemic proportions worldwide. Its prevalence is fast spreading to younger age groups too, so much so that now childhood obesity has been identified as a significant health concern. Over one half of adult American population is over weight or obese. Its highest prevalence has been found out to be among the 25 to 35 year age group. But the problem is common across all age groups. The healthcare costs of obesity run into hundreds of billions of dollars.

Obesity is a major cardiovascular risk factor. It also directly contributes to high blood pressure, diabetes and high cholesterol levels. Thus the cardiovascular risk of obesity is much higher than the risk associated with any other singular risk factor. Obesity causes lung disease, stroke, arthritis, depression and many forms of cancers. It is causes infertility in young women. The full list of maladies caused by obesity is very long. This list includes obstructive sleep apnea, carpal tunnel syndrome, deep venous thrombosis, leg ulcers, varicose veins, leg swelling, infections, liver disease, back injury and pancreatitis. Obesity makes even simple surgical procedures quite risky and complicated. Surgeons find it technically hard to work when the body-anatomy is so distorted by the excess fat deposits. The complications of surgery in the obese include non-healing of surgical wounds and even reopening of the closed wounds. Obesity increases the risk of wound infections as well as lung infections after surgery. The obese are more prone to developing clots in the legs and in lungs after surgery. Due to these complications mortality of surgery could become very high. This is why some times surgeons refuse to operate on the obese patients.

Obesity is almost always linked to high blood pressure, diabetes (or early diabetes) and high cholesterol levels. Though obesity has been identified as an independent risk factor for heart disease, the bad combination of the above mentioned three risk factors with obesity makes it extremely dangerous. The exact mechanism by which obesity acts as an independent risk factor for heart disease is still uncertain. Its ill effects on the inner lining of the arteries may be a major factor contributing to this risk.

Weight gain and obesity is the result of relative or absolute physical inactivity and excess eating. Genetics play a big role in the development of obesity. The latter includes intake of excess calories and fat that is abundant in cheaper and more conveniently obtained foods. Thus obesity is a life style disorder perpetuated by socioeconomic and environmental factors. Obesity and excess weight are most prevalent amongst women, the poor and the ethnic minorities. Lack of knowledge and financial constraints are the major contributors to this trend in its distribution. Rarely obesity can be caused by some hormonal disorders such thyroid hormone inactivity or excess of natural steroids. Such situations should be treated medically.

Obesity has a scientific classification dependent on the body weight and height. This is based on the concept of the body mass index or BMI. BMI can be calculated by dividing ones weight in kilograms by the squared height in meters. A normal or desirable BMI is between 19 and 24 (a BMI below 18 signifies under nutrition). A BMI between 25 and 29.9 is classified as "over weight". Any BMI above 30 is considered obese. Waist circumference of more than 40 inches in men and more than 35 inches in women too suggest obesity. These values have been associated with increased risk of illness and death.

Why lose weight?

Many disorders that the obese suffer can be cured or improved simply by losing weight. Even a small amount of weight loss is known to be hugely beneficial to health. Despite the proven health benefits, statistics say that less than 50% of surveyed doctors claim to promote weight loss among their patients. Ills of obesity and benefits of losing weight have been acknowledged and documented in the medic al literature from the east since thousands of years ago. Ancient Ayurvedic manuscripts from India discuss the multiple associated sicknesses of obesity and highlight its link with heart disease. In the modern era it was the life insurance companies that first observed the relation ship between losing weight and improved health. Obesity is now well recognized as a complex medical condition with high mortality. A large trial that studied close to 30 000 overweight women reported that planned weight loss of more than 20 lbs decreased mortality of the population by almost 25%.

In addition weight loss is known to reduce the body's resistance to the activity of the hormone insulin. Resistance to insulin gives rise to diabetes. In a well-publicized Swedish study into obesity, researchers observed complete cure of diabetes among those who achieved significant weight loss after gastric bypass surgery. Obesity has also been associated with elevated blood levels of C reactive protein that is identified as an independent risk factor for coronary artery disease. C reactive protein levels go down with weight loss and this brings about further protection from heart disease.

All diseases of the arteries including coronary arteries originate from malfunctioning of the inner lining of the arteries. This lining is made up of a single layer of cells that covers the inner surface of all arteries in the body. When this lining or the endothelium is defective or malfunctioning cholesterol plaques build up and gradually narrow the arteries compromising blood flow through them. Obesity is a direct risk factor for endothelial dysfunction. Weight loss is found out to be beneficial to the endothelium.

Compared to the scale of the problem not enough scientific research work has been carried out into the prevention and treatment of obesity. This deficiency is also well apparent in the efforts at public education and awareness promotion on obesity. Standard means of obesity management can take several different forms. These include lifestyle and diet management, behavioral or psychological therapy, medical therapy and surgical therapy. None of these treatment methods are mutually exclusive. Often the management plans for obesity are multi-disciplinary and multi-pronged.

The ideal strategy should be decided upon by you and your doctor after giving much thought. No strategy would be successful without your unreserved corporation and willingness to comply fully. After all, the onus is going to be on you to change your lifestyle and spend the necessary resources and time on obtaining treatment. Therefore any planning should be preceded by clear identification of practical short term and realistic long-term goals and a pledge to commit to such goals. It is equally important to harness as much support in every way possible from your immediate social network of family and friends.

Diet

Once the basic and essential knowledge on nutrition is acquired you are ready to look at you own diet to see what food is bad and has to be stopped or changed or substituted. The hardest aspect of diet therapy is change: initiating practical change and maintaining such change. No change is practical or conceivable without a strong desire and a compelling motivation. You and your doctor with other resource personnel should work together with equal enthusiasm to lay this mental groundwork. Eliciting the support of your close social network is invaluable both for overseeing and for encouraging you to make and maintain change. In his regard you should solicit the support of your family members, friends and colleagues at work. Controlling the portions you eat and the frequency at which you eat are as important as avoiding high calorie, high carbohydrate and high fat food that contribute to weight gain.

Attempts at weight loss are challenging and often end up in failure. Weight loss therapy is expensive be it life style oriented, medical or surgical. Maintenance of weight loss once it is achieved is difficult too. But gains of losing weight in terms of health and quality of life are tremendously significant. Therefore these gains should be upheld and reinforced as factors of motivation.

Due to the prevalence of the condition there are many options available as weight-loss remedies out there. Given the sheer number of the different options it is often unnerving and confusing to decide on the best and the most suitable. In addition caution should be exercised with the adoption of some methods because of the potential for serious harm and at times even death. Therefore the best way to start is to discuss your plans for weight loss with your doctor. Any level of excess weight should be first addressed with diet therapy. The fundamentals of diet therapy include education, review and change. No diet therapy plan would be successful without your knowing the concepts of good and bad nutrition. Learning about different constituents of a your diet, the concept of calorie intake and the details on fat etc should lay the ground work of your diet management plan.

Obesity is the results of consuming more calories than you spend each day. Therefore to reverse the situation you should spend more calories than you eat. And once the healthy weight range is achieved, daily calorie intake should be adjusted to balance the calorie expenditure. Reducing food intake is the best and most effective way to lose weight fast. However to maintain weight loss you should increase calorie expenditure by increasing physical activity.

Basic daily energy requirement of an average size (60kg) woman is approximately 1400kcalories. For an average size man (80kg) it would be 1800kcalories. So according to your weight you can determine how many calories would make you maintain your weight at its current level by balancing your calorie intake to the basic calorie expenditure. To lose weight you should take in less calories than the required amount for maintenance. Adding physical activity to the equation would make you lose more calories. Thus you can workout how much you should eat and how much you should exercise to bring about a negative calorie balance that would facilitate weight loss. This is the governing principle of lifestyle intervention for weight loss. If lifestyle interventions, despite strict compliance do not effect in causing a weight loss of at least 5 kilograms in the first three months, you should discuss additional strategies and other options with your doctor.

Physical exercise

The other integral aspect of life style therapy for obesity is physical exercise. Researchers have demonstrated that moderate aerobic exercise even at least 30 minutes a day is useful in effecting tangible weight loss. While aerobic exercise such as walking, jogging and swimming help burn excess calories other forms exercise such as light-weight training and yoga too has been found out to be effective in the battle to lose weight. Yoga helps develop mental concentration and build up the psychological conditioning necessary for compliance with the weight loss program. The stress relieving aspects of exercise helps to over come the craving for more food. In addition incorporation of exercise such as yoga and pilates makes the whole process more enjoyable as well as fashionable. According to the results of some well-controlled trials practicing yoga can result in significant weight loss. The other important aspect of exercise is that its effects could be cumulative even if performed for short periods of time on separate occasions over the course of the day. Thus when the options necessitating physical exertion is chosen over the more automated option, one can perform a good deal of physical activity without having to take time to work out. For example, if you to take the stairs instead of the elevator, wash dishes manually instead of using the washing machine and take strolls instead of using the car for transportation involving short distances you will spend enough calories to exceed your calorie intake.

For optimal and long lasting results diet option should always be combined with the physical exercise option.

Drug therapy

If you are clinically obese (BMI of over 30) or if you are over weight and suffer from medical conditions given rise to by your excess weight or if life style changes have not brought about anticipated weight loss you and your doctor should discuss the option of medical therapy. Your doctor will give you all the information necessary regarding the medical options available today. Your should keep in mind that these treatment options can have side effect that can at times be quite harmful. Therefore this option should be taken with close supervision and follow up of your doctor. Drug therapy should always be accompanied by the life style changes of diet modification and regular physical exercise. It should be borne in mind that drug therapy cannot by any means cure obesity. The drug options currently available include Ephedrine, Sibutramine (Meridia), Phentermine and Orilstat (Xenical). There are other agents being developed or pending approval from authorities for public use.

The effects of the former three agents mimic the activity of body's sympathetic nervous system. These drugs act by either increasing body's resting energy expenditure through generating heat or by causing early satiety thus preventing excess eating. You should however watch for the side effects of dry mouth, constipation, tremor and difficulty with sleeping when taking these drugs. Research has shown that combination of ephedrine with caffeine could bring about more effective weight loss than ephedrine alone. Similar effects have been observed with the use of a Chinese herbal agent called Ma Huang, when taken in combination with caffeine. However herbal agents such as Ma Huang have not been thoroughly tested for short and long term safety therefore should not be taken without consulting your doctor.

Sibutramine and some other anti obesity drugs can affect the activity of your heart. They cause your blood pressure and your heart rate to go up. Therefore it is not advisable to take these drugs if you have heart disease. Also you should not take these drugs if you are on certain antidepressants because of the possibility of major drug interactions.

Orilstat or xenical acts by inhibiting the action of an enzyme that helps digest fat in your diet. It acts mainly in your intestines and therefore only a very little of it actually gets absorbed into your body. Randomized controlled studies have confirmed that treatment with orilstat can cause significant weight loss. As a result of orilstat therapy stool fat content rises significantly. Non- digested fat is responsible for the side effects of oirlstat treatment that includes intestinal cramps, intestinal gas, incontinence and diarrhea. It can also reduce the absorption of fat-soluble vitamins such as vitamins A, D and E.

There are other drugs that have shown great promise as effective anti-obesity agents. Leptin is one such agent. Leptin is a protein type chemical compound naturally produced in the body's fat tissue. Absence of leptin or the resistance to its activity leads to significant obesity. When leptin is given to those that lack it, their food intake and consequently the body weight go down. But if you have resistance to the activity of leptin in your body, this weight loss would not come about. Many obese people have been identified as having a genetically mediated resistance to the action of leptin. They have high levels of leptin their blood. Treating these people with extra-high doses of leptin can some times help cause weight loss. However leptin therapy is not yet approved as a treatment for obesity in the US.

Two other protein like substances (peptides) have been identified as beneficial treatment for obesity. These are glucagon like peptide and peptide YY. Both these agent act by decreasing your food intake.

Green tea has an effect of generating heat inside the body. Thus this may show promise as a safe herbal alternative for tablet treatment.

Surgery

Surgical option is reserved for those who are extremely obese with a BMI of over 40. If you have obesity related medical complications even with a BMI of 35-39.9 you may benefit form surgery. Surgery has been shown to be an effective means of treating extreme obesity with good long-term results. Surgery to reduce obesity is called bariatric surgery and involves surgical resection of the stomach and the intestines to limit the amount of food eaten and absorbed into the body. You should ensure that you are operated by a well-qualified and experienced surgeon since obesity surgery can lead to dangerous complications in the hands of the unwary.

Chapter 5

Doctor, am I also at risk?

I was introduced to Martin by a friend of mine. He was 35 years old, physically fit and with no health problems. But he had a very serious concern. His father has had a heart attack at the age of 46. He has had no known coronary risk factor. According to Martin his father was slim, never smoked, had no high blood pressure, no diabetes and no problems with his cholesterol levels. He has been very active physically, regularly jogging and swimming. "My father was like a model of good health, and then he gets a heart attacks out of the blue" Martin claimed. His tone was that of disappointment and amazement. Then he asked me the critical question. "Doc what is my risk of getting a heart attack? He went on "what am I to do now"?

Martin's dilemma is neither new nor unique. I have encountered so many with similar stories and questions. Incidentally just about a week prior to my meeting Martin I happened to meet another man whose situation mirrored that of Martin. He was David a 40-year-old commercial airline pilot with a strong family history similar to that of Martin. He was referred to me by an internist colleague with the exact question "what should we do?" Unfortunately there is no single answer to this question. I told Martin just as I did to David that he certainly was at risk. But how much of a risk he was at? I could not say. Is there anything that Martin, David or I could do? Yes. There are many things that we could do hopefully to prevent heart diseased. First thing to do in this situation is to estimate the relative risk of each individual of developing heart disease. The next step would be to choose the best course of action to minimize the risk. But each action should be evaluated on its own merit to see whether it would benefit in each individual's context.

There are screening tests done in clinical medicine to assess whether individuals without symptoms have early evidence of a certain disease. Screening tests are useful in diseases that can be treated more effectively if diagnosed early. Screening tests are done in individuals at a certain risk of developing the disease condition of interest. David and Martin were without any symptoms. Is there any thing that can be gained by doing screening tests for coronary artery disease in any of these two men? Screening inappropriately can mean an unnecessary expense. The more unnecessary tests you perform the higher the impact of it on the over all health care budget. Such excess expenditure results in health care becoming more and more expensive. Doing a diagnostic test with no real practical value can also generate unnecessary psychological stress in you. Reliability of a screening test to diagnose a disease is dependent on how likely you are to develop the disease. This phenomenon is called the "pre test probability".

To prevent unnecessary testing of people and to ensure right people are screened, health authorities have laid down guidelines for the medical practitioners. Guidelines say that men with no symptoms but with two or more coronary risk factors may benefit from screening for coronary disease. 10% of people belonging to this category are believed to have coronary artery disease. Another group of people that would benefit from screening is those whose jobs involve the responsibility and safety of many people. Airline pilots, truck drivers, train drivers are some such individuals. A sudden heart attack in such an individual while at work would jeopardize not only his or her life but also of hundreds of others. Then there are those who decide to start physical exercise after prolonged periods of relative physical inactivity. Since unusual physical exertion can trigger a heart attack in a risk prone individual, it is strongly advised that these individuals be cleared of any risk by screening prior to commencing physical exercise.

There was enough reason for me to screen David the airline pilot for heart disease. But for Martin, I believed it was not necessary at this stage. First I went on to check the blood pressure, blood glucose levels and blood cholesterol levels in both individuals. Everything was within normal limits. Family histories of premature heart disease and male gender were strong risk factors both these individual had. Therefore I could not dismiss their risks of early heart disease without further testing. High risk necessitates lifestyle intervention or treatment. If you are at high risk you may still benefit from treatment in the prevention of heart disease. Many advocate treatment of high-risk individuals with a statin drug even if cholesterol levels are within the normal range. There is increasing evidence to suggest that the traditional risk factor profile of male gender, middle age, smoking, diabetes, high blood pressure, high cholesterol levels and a family history accounts only for a part of the picture. Research has revealed many more factors that would make an individual to be at risk of developing heart disease. Some such factors can be tested for while others not. But most such novel coronary risk factors are still at the level of experimentation that it would be a considerable period of time before testing for such factors are made available widely. I had to keep in mind that both David and Martin may harbor such novel risk factors that may have predisposed their fathers to have heart attacks.

Scientists have been, over a considerable period of time trying to find the association of such novel and putative risk factors and heart disease. While some factors that were thought to increase the risk of heart disease proved not to do so and fell by the ways side others remained to be tested further. One such factor that showed promise as a risk factor and endured the rigors of scientific testing is the CRP level in your blood. CRP stands for C-Reactive Protein. This is a chemical compound released by the body when it fights against an insult or an injury or when mounting an inflammatory response. CRP concentration in blood is elevated to very high levels when you have an infection or a condition like arthritis or even after a heart attack. It can be checked with a blood test that is available at many laboratories.

CRP levels

Highly sensitive CRP level has been recognized as an independent marker of coronary risk. You can check the CRP level by performing a relatively cheap blood test. Experts have recommended that CRP be tested in those who have an intermediate risk of developing coronary artery disease in the long term. Thus it should be done after assessing the presence of more direct markers of coronary risk and establishing the absence thereof. It is not recommended as a population based screening method. It is advised to be done in duplicate, one fasting and the other non-fasting, within a two week's interval. A h-CRP level of <1 mg/L is considered low risk and between 1-3 mg/L is considered average risk. Any value >3 mg/L is high risk. This test should be done in the absence of any other obvious inflammation or infection to prevent interference. Anyone with a high h-CRP level should bc considered as being at high risk of developing heart disease. They seem to benefit from statin therapy due to the anti-inflammatory action of it.

Homocysteine

Those who suffer from the genetic condition called homocysteinuria develop coronary heart disease at a very young age. Homocysteinurics have a defect in the pathway of metabolizing or breaking down amino acids in the body due to the inability to produce certain enzymes. But doctors noticed that some times even those who do not have homocysteinuria have elevated levels of homocyeteine in the blood. They argued that just like the homocysteinurics those who have higher levels of homocysteine in the blood run an increased risk of developing heart disease. Many scientific experiments subsequently confirmed this hypothesis.

In a recent article published in the Annals of Internal medicine an Israeli group reported that high serum homocysteine levels in those who have had a heart attack already, predicts the likelihood of getting more heart attacks in the future. They went on to say that high homocysteine levels also predicted an increased risk of death in these individuals. This risk prediction was real no matter what other risk factors were present and it was found out to be independent of the severity of the narrowing in their coronary arteries.

Homocysteine level is not checked routinely in the assessment of patients at high risk of developing heart disease. It may be justified in those who seem to be at risk even without any evidence to the presence of the more conventional risk factors. Regular supplementation of folic acid and pyridoxine (vitamin B6) is known to reduce the homocysteine level in the blood.

Genetics

There is no secret that genetics play a significant role in the development of coronary heart disease. The fact that this disease runs in families is ample testimony to this effect. It is believed that environmental factors such as life style, diet and physical activity can turn on or turn off, these genes to increase or decrease your risk of getting heart disease. Scientists have identified many genes that are considered to be associated with coronary heart disease. However coronary artery disease is considered a "multigenic" disorder where multiple genes play a role in causing the risk. Still there is no genetic test that has been discovered to screen populations to identify those at risk. There is intense scientific research taking place to "hunt" for the "heart disease gene". Scientists are studying the genetic make up of those who have bad coronary arteries to compare it with that of those who are healthy to identify the genetic factors of difference in the two groups. It is expected that such research will eventually lead to the development of tests to identify he high risk genetic make up in the risk prone individuals. With further advancement of technology we can anticipate that one day, gene therapy would be available as treatment against heart disease.

Despite having a normal coronary risk factor profile apart from a strong family history I did not want to let Martin go without making it absolutely clear that his risk of developing heart disease is minimal at this stage. So I checked his ultra sensitive CRP level and homocysteine level. His CRP level was high and the homocysteine level was normal. Still I did not want to start him on a statin drug straightaway. Instead I advised him to change his life style to a heart friendly one with regular exercise and diet management. I plan to recheck his CRP level in another three months. If it is still high I will commence him on a statin drug to prevent him from falling victim to heart disease prematurely.

But for David I decided to take a different approach because of his occupation. I wanted to be absolutely sure that he did not have any evidence of heart disease prior to commencing him on preventive therapy or discharging him without any therapy. So I did an exercise stress test on him to look for the presence of any coronary disease. Exercise stress test is a screening test for heart disease. His exercise stress test was negative. It was reassuring but did not give me information to decide on commencing or not commencing preventative therapy. Next I went on to test his ultra sensitive CRP level and homocysteine level. Both tests came back as normal. Nevertheless there is no way I could say that he is not at risk of developing premature heart disease because of his positive family history. Therefore I advised him to change his life style to heart friendly one. I plan to follow up David at six monthly intervals.

There are instances where screening tests become important in patients who already have some symptoms of heart disease despite belong to a traditionally low risk population. Vladislav is one such individual that was referred to me by a family practitioner. He is a 42-year old diplomat who lived and worked at the UN headquarters in New York. He was involved with the work at his country's mission to the UN. In addition his duties involved working with the UN security council. His job was "highly stressful" he told me during my conversation with him. Since of late he has been experiencing tightness in the middle of his chest particularly when he felt stressed. My assessment revealed that he had no other coronary risk factor apart from being over weight. Because his symptoms could suggest coronary heart disease I referred him for an exercise stress test. The stress results said "negative for significant coronary artery disease". On most patients I would be happy with a negative exercise stress test to discharge a patient without any further investigation. But in the case of Vladislav I wanted to be absolutely sure. Best way to find out the real nature of his coronary arteries would be to do an angiogram. But without a compelling indication and in the presence of a negative stress test I was reluctant to perform an invasive test with rare but potential complications. I wanted another test that is non-invasive and relatively inexpensive to comfortably rule out the presence of coronary artery disease prior to deciding on an angiogram.

I referred him for "EBCT" or electron beam computed tomography test. The test came back positive with a calcium score of 450. This result was very suggestive of some serious narrowing of coronary arteries. Since there was enough justification now as the next step I performed an angiogram on Vladislav and my suspicion was confirmed. He had a significant narrowing in one of the large coronary arteries. I could open this artery without much difficulty with a balloon. Then I placed a new drug coated stent and completed the procedure. Vladislav still had to minimize his coronary risk factors to prevent the development of further narrowing of coronary arteries in the future. I educated him on life style changes that are necessary and commenced him on a diet and exercise program to reduce his excess weight. I advised him to start yoga exercise too once or twice a week with the objective of relieving stress. Vladislav's is an example where exercise stress test alone may not conclusively exclude one's coronary risk. It is good that there are more tests available today to further assess patients with an intermediate risk before testing further with invasive tests or discharging altogether with no treatment.

EBCT scan

EBCT scan or the electron beam computed tomography scan has become a popular mode of investigation of one's risk of heart disease. Despite its popularity it has not found uniform acceptance among all cardiologists. But it is important to examine what it offers and what role it has to play in modern cardiology given the popularity it seem to enjoy among the general public.

EBCT is a rapid scanning procedure that is entirely non-invasive and very low-risk. It takes x-ray pictures of the heart, particularly the coronary arteries and measures the amount of calcium deposited in the walls of these arteries. Once the picture is taken it analyzes and quantifies the amount of coronary calcium according to a scoring system. This score is reported as a coronary risk score called the "calcium score". It is considered that higher the ones calcium score is the higher the risk of heart disease. This is essentially a test for those who do not have any symptoms of heart disease and those who are not known to be at very high risk of heart disease. Those who have some symptoms to suggest heart disease too may benefit by EBCT testing, particularly if the exercise stress test is inconclusive. Calcium score helps to make treatment decisions in those who are at some risk or at questionable risk of heart disease.

Atherosclerotic plaques that deposit in the coronary arteries contain calcium. Normal coronary arteries do not have such calcium deposits. So the basis of EBCT is to detect such calcium deposits and estimate indirectly the presence or absence of coronary artery disease. Studies done in animals as well as in human have shown that the degree of calcium deposition can indicate the severity of the disease. However it is important to note that calcium score cannot give a direct assessment of the degree of narrowing of the coronary arteries due to the plaques. But the researchers say that a high calcium score, particularly above 150, warns of likely narrowing of the arteries. This is very important in those who fail to experience symptoms despite having narrowed coronary arteries like those suffering from diabetes.

On the other hand a normal EBCT scan (of zero score) or a low calcium score is said to predict safety from any coronary heart disease for the next 5 to 15 years. However just like anything else in medicine EBCT or the calcium score is not 100% fool proof. There are anecdotal reports of patients having had massive heart attacks even after being cleared by an EBCT scan with a low calcium score. A calcium score of more than 400 is considered high and of significant concern. In the relevant studied this score has been associated with the presence of significant narrowing of coronary arteries and positive stress tests.

I recently tested a 34-year-old man named Paul who presented to me with very high blood cholesterol levels. He had no other known coronary risk factors. I had to make a decision with regards to prescribing him cholesterol-lowering tablets. I did not want to expose him to a drug and burden him with the cost of paying for it perhaps for the rest of his life, without compelling evidence to support my decision. So I did an EBCT scan on him. His calcium score was high and I started him on the tablet. Evidence from studies suggests that I can follow patients like Paul over time by repeated EBCT scan to assess their disease progression

Doctors have found out that EBCT scan can be used as a safe way of monitoring how patients respond to cholesterol lowering treatment. They have noticed that with the lowering of total cholesterol levels and particularly the LDL cholesterol level many individuals showed a gradual reduction in the calcium score. On the other hand those that fail to show a reduction in the calcium score or those that show an increase can have their drug doses increased and other measures taken to prevent the progression of their heart disease.

Concept of the endothelium and the cardiac risk

Endothelium is the inner covering of all hollow body organ s including the blood vessels. Since it covers a large area, it is considered to be the largest organ in the body. It is similar to a skin over the inner surfaces of the body. The major contributor to coronary artery disease is the disorders of the endothelium. Heart attacks happen when the arteries that supply blood to the heart gets blocked. This blocking of the coronary arteries is the end result of progressive poor health and damage to the endothelium covering the blood vessels that supply the heart. Same phenomenon applies to the brain too. Strokes happen when an artery supplying a part of the brain gets blocked off. This too is due diseased state of the endothelium of these arteries.

Since of late major focus in the research into heart disease and stroke have been focused on the function and good health of the endothelium. Statin drugs have been identified as contributing to the stability and the health of the endothelium. This effect goes beyond its cholesterol reducing properties in ameliorating the risk of heart disease. Just as we take great care to look after our skin to maintain physical appearance, it is important to look after the endothelium, or the inner skin to maintain good health and longevity. Just like bad lifestyle factors such as exposure to pollutants and harsh sunlight can damage your skin your life style factors of bad diet, stress and physical inactivity can damage your endothelium. Diet rich in fresh fruits, vegetables, nut, legumes and low in calories and fat is endothelium friendly. Regular physical exercise also helps the preservation of the endothelium. Practices such as yoga and meditation that brings about stress relief too are known to benefit the endothelium. Protecting your endothelium is a prime objective in your fight against heart disease.

Stress and Psychological factors

Deborah was an investment banker who was brought to our hospital with severe chest pain one Monday morning. When I reviewed her in the ER I realized that she was having a bad heart attack. When I examined her EKG my suspicion was confirmed. We quickly took her to the catheterization laboratory and opened the blocked coronary that was causing her heart attack. The operation was straight-forward and successful. She did not suffer much damage to her heart and subsequently made a swift recovery. Though every thing went well and Deborah was discharged home after two days there was some thing unusual about her case. Until the day she had the heart attack she was perfectly healthy. She was slim, fit and truly glamorous. She was a successful career woman, a wife and a mother of three teen-aged daughters. She exercise regularly and never smoked. She ate healthy food and led an exemplary life style. She did not even have a family history of heart disease. It is rare for women like Deborah with no known coronary risk factor to develop heart disease at her age. Most women of Deborah's age that present with heart attacks either smoke, obese or have diabetes.

Talking to Deborah after the catheterization shed some light to the mystery of Deborah's heart attack. At the moment when she first experienced tightness in her chest she was addressing a meeting. It was no ordinary meeting or routine engagement. It was a meeting that was to decide the fate of her company for which a take over bid has been launched by a rival company. She as the core-director was against the move and there was a chance that she would lose her position if the company were to be taken over. She had worked tirelessly over the previous few months to change the way things were heading with her company. It has been a very stressful period. She noticed that she lost her temper often. She was always edgy and snapped at anybody for the slightest reason. She has had fights even with her husband and the daughters. The usually peaceful household disturbed. The worries at her work place kept Deborah oblivious to the fact that her own stress was consuming her health and her personal life. And it all culminated with her sustaining the heart attack that fateful Monday morning.
Before her discharge from the hospital, I had to discuss the important issue of stress relief with Deborah. It was not straight-forward like giving advice on changing the diet or taking up physical exercise. Stressors of her life and especially her career were beyond the control of both of us. I could only advice her on measures to combat the effect of such stress. There is no drug treatment for stress. I advised her and her husband to take a holiday to start with. I also advised her to find a qualified yoga teacher and start up on a yoga program. I did not want to refer her to a psychologist since I knew that she was not having psychological problems. Like Deborah many fall victim to heart disease due to stress and strife in life. The effect of stress and stress prone personality on heart health has been well described in medicine.

There is enough evidence to associate high mental stress with heart disease. It is another adverse life style factor of the modern era together with unhealthy diet and physical inactivity that promote heart disease. The association of stress with heart disease has been largely anecdotal and casual. In a similar manner benefit of stress reduction to heart health too has been speculative, however, with good evidence. The association of coronary artery disease and the so called "high strung" and "high stressed" type A personality has been long recognized. Behavioral traits of anger, rage, hostility, competitiveness and cynicism are associated with the vulnerable type A personality. But later tests failed to substantiate this putative risk and therefore many doctors today dismiss the importance of stress as a direct cardiac risk factor.

Many observations have linked highly stressful circumstances with the triggering of heart attacks and also sudden death due to cardiac arrest. In some studies "emotional upheaval" has been identified as the most common trigger of heart attacks and sudden death. High stress can cause your blood pressure and pulse rate to rise very significantly thus placing a high burden on your heart. It is also known to increase the propensity of your blood to clot more. Both factors in combination create ideal circumstances for a massive heart attack in anyone who has narrowing of coronary arteries.

A large study called the "Atherosclerosis risk in communities trial" that studied close to 13000 men and women for the relationship between anger and heart disease showed that subjects with normal blood pressure and who are easily angered or constantly angry had a high risk of heart disease and death compared to those who were not easily angered. Anger and related behavioral traits have been associated with early onset of heart disease in other observational studies.

Evidence is also accumulating that links long-term stress with the development of coronary artery disease. Stress is considered to contribute to the development of coronary disease by triggering the release of unhealthy neurological and hormonal factors that over a long period of time can damage the endothelium lining the inner surface of the arteries. Such damage causes the deposition of cholesterol and the build up of plaques in the inner wall of arteries that eventually cause their narrowing. In addition psychological stress causes you to smoke, eat more (particularly high calorie, high fat food) and causes your blood pressure to go up – all factors that damage the endothelium and cause heart disease.

Doctors have long observed that heart attacks and cardiac arrests happen more frequently in the early hours of the day. This has been confirmed beyond argument by large observational studies. Your blood pressure usually peaks around mid morning. In addition there are reports to suggest that most heart attacks happen on Mondays compared to other days of the week. Early hours of the day and the first day of the week are undoubtedly the more stressful times of the modern life style. Another interesting observation is the high incidence of heart attacks and sudden death in the winter months compared to the summer. Supporting these observations are the increased incidence of heart attacks and cardiac arrests reported in communities in the aftermath of major catastrophes such as bomb blasts, earthquakes and other disasters where collective stress levels go up.

These time and circumstances related difference in the incidence of heart attacks has not been observed in those suffering from diabetes. This may be due to the fact that diabetic individuals fail to mount neurological and hormonal responses to stressful situations like those without diabetes due to the diabetes associated nerve disease. This fact further confirms the interplay of stress and neurological and hormonal factors in triggering heart attacks and causing sudden death.

Though not recognized widely psychological factors seem to be directly associated with the long term development of narrowing in the coronary arteries as well with the triggering of heart attacks and causing sudden death. Due to these reasons I believe that stress reduction should be incorporated to the life style modification therapy in the prevention and also treatment of heart disease.

I saw Deborah and her husband in my office one moth later. She appeared well and more relaxed. She told me that she decided to quit her job after giving it much thought. She was making preparation to join a university in an academic position where she thought the stress levels were low. She has commenced yoga and was enjoying it. Her physical examination was unremarkable and she was essentially well. However I advised her to avoid stressful circumstances as much as she could because stress remained her main cardiac risk factor.

Chapter 6

Eat well, live well - Diet and the heart

Nutrition and health have a direct and a close relationship. What we eat can make us sick or healthy. This is by far the fact when it comes to heart disease and other disorders and conditions that are risk factors for heart disease. Heart disease is called a lifestyle disorder because lifestyle factors including the diet have a direct contribution to the development of heart disease. Just as an unhealthy and unplanned diet contributes to heart disease, a planned and a healthy diet can contribute to the prevention of heart disease. In this chapter we will consider the elements of our diet that may contribute to the development of heart disease or risk factors thereof and examine the ways we can make the right changes and right choices to make our diet healthy. A large volume of scientific work has been carried out looking into the key nutritional factors associated with heart disease both in negative as well as positive ways. As more and more work is being done and new discoveries are made the knowledge of the relationship between different food types and heart disease seem to evolve rapidly.

Our diet is mainly made up of fat, carbohydrates, proteins, minerals, vitamins, water and undigestable material such as fiber. Whatever food we may eat in whatever form or preparation, can finally be broken down to the above elements. So it is easier to examine the diet's effect on heart disease by focusing on the effect of each of its constituents on heart disease and heart health.

Diet and dieting have been brandied about in the healthcare literature so much that at times it ends up creating confusion than being helpful. But the importance of dietary planning in the prevention and control of heart disease cannot be emphasized more. Dietary planning will help lose weight, control cholesterol levels, control blood sugar levels in the diabetics and help blood pressure lowering. Healthy diet is known to benefit not only in the prevention of heart disease but also in the prevention of disorders of other organs and also cancers.

It is not too difficult to plan a healthy diet if you understand the basic principles of healthy nutrition. Avoiding excess is the fundamental premise of healthy eating. Eating in smaller portions so as to satisfy your appetite should be the main objective. Any excess to that what satisfies your hunger should be deliberately avoided. Just as the quantity, the quality or the content of your food should be planned and controlled. High carbohydrate and high fat containing food should be avoided as much as possible and kept to a minimum when consumed. Fresh fruits, fresh vegetables, whole grains and food containing high amounts of fiber should be consumed more.

Just as acquiring new knowledge, it is important to put into practice the knowledge thus gained in changing life style and diet. The changes should be made with a clear objective, a vision and a set goal. The change should be made gradually with step-by-step progression. The change should be made in a planned and systematic way. Finally the change should be made on a collective basis with the consensus and the support of your spouse and significant others in your family.

First step in the process of planning on healthy eating is to obtain more knowledge on what is good and what is not good to eat and the reasons behind such categorization. The next step is to examine your current dietary patterns to identify which items are not so wholesome and what habits need changing. Once this initial assessment is done it is easy to substitute, reduce and increase the different types of food accordingly. A firm resolution and a commitment will enable consistent practice of good and healthy dietary habits.

Calories and calorie counting

Energy value, the fat content and the fat type in the food are the most important aspects to watch for in planning and controlling your diet. If you consume more energy than needed for the activities of daily living and body's natural function it gets stored in body as energy deposits. Most energy deposits take the form of fat eventually. This high-energy food consumed more than the daily requirement leads to fat deposition, weight gain and obesity.

Calorie counting involves assessing the energy value of the food you eat. Calorie is a measure of energy. Energy requirements are in fact calculated in kilocalories (kilocalorie = 1000 calories). In the popular conversation the terms calorie and kilocalorie are used interchangeably. The food we eat is oxidized or burned in the cells to generate energy for our day-to-day activities as well for life sustaining activities at the level of the cells. These activities at the level of the cell are collectively called metabolic activities. Metabolic activities essentially involve the general house keeping of the body and the incidentals. Carbohydrates, proteins and fats in our diet can be broken down to produce energy. Far more energy can be generated from the burning of fat than of carbohydrates and proteins. So therefore fat has more calories than carbohydrates and proteins when considered in equal amounts. Energy consumed in excess of what is necessary for expenditure for body activity is transformed predominantly to fat and is deposited in the body. This leads to weight gain and obesity. Increased fat deposits and associated obesity lead to excess levels of fat and cholesterol (which is a form of fat) in the blood. Fat also increases your blood sugar levels and your blood pressure. Increased blood sugar levels can lead to diabetes.

It is important to have a basic understanding of the calorie content of different food types. It is also of equal importance to have a basic understanding of the fat content of the different food types. Many processed food types have labels with a description of the nutritional content in the form of different food elements in their proportions such as carbohydrates, fats, and protein content per unit weight or per serving. It also states the total energy value per unit weight or per serving.

Best way to understand how much calories one needs per day is to know how much calories are needed to sustain life at rest (with no or minimal physical activity) and know the calorie expenditure of different activities. The total of calories needed at rest and the total activities should be balanced by the estimated calorie content of all the food you eat in a day.

Calorie expenditure of different activities (kilocalories per half hour)

Sitting	40
Gardening	110
Golf	100
Walking (4mph)	150
Swimming	150
Bicycling (10mph)	195
Tennis	210
Jogging (5mph)	265
Running (8mph)	360

To lose 1 lb of your body weight you should consume 500 calories less than your total daily calorie expenditure.

Recommended calorie intake per day (resting)

Average size female	1400
Average size male	1800

Fat and cholesterol

Fat consumed in the unhealthy forms and in excess is contributory in a very significant manner to the development of heart disease and the cardiac risk factors of excess blood cholesterol levels and obesity. Fat contributes the most amount of energy per unit mass of all dietary components. 1 gram of fat can generate 9 calories. It is recommended that less than 30% of the daily calorie intake be from the fat in our food.

The food we eat contains different types of fats that behave in your body in different ways. Some forms of fat are more harmful to the heart than others. Meanwhile there are some other forms of fat that may behave in a manner that would promote heart health. The different types of fats include saturated fats, mono unsaturated fats, polyunsaturated fats and trans fats.

Cholesterol is a form of fat found in the blood and tissues of our body. While cholesterol can be taken in with food we eat, most cholesterol in our body is made within the body from the fatty acids we absorb from the fats we eat in our diet. Cholesterol in right levels is necessary for the healthy function of the body and for the synthesis of different hormones. Cholesterol when found in excess can lead to heart disease. There are different forms of cholesterol circulating in the blood. Some cholesterol types when in excess can be harmful to the body whilst other forms may be beneficial.

Good and bad cholesterol

There are three major form of cholesterol in the blood stream as I have discussed before. You may remember that hey include HDL cholesterol, LDL cholesterol and triglycerides. LDL cholesterol and triglycerides are considered the bad forms of cholesterol. The atherosclerotic plaques that cause the narrowing of blood vessels contain high levels of LDL cholesterol. LDL cholesterol is known to promote plaque deposition. In addition they cause plaques to damage (rupture) thus causing clot formation within the already narrowed arteries causing them to block off completely - the mechanism by which heart attacks and strokes often happen. Triglycerides too contribute to the deposition and the build up of cholesterol plaques. When found in very high levels triglycerides can cause dangerous inflammation of the pancreas. The "good" cholesterol or HDL cholesterol causes the "bad" LDL cholesterol to be removed from blood stream. Thus they help reduce the deposition of plaques in the arteries.

When the doctor measures blood cholesterol levels it is tested after a 12 hour (usually overnight) fast. This is believed to give an accurate estimation of the usual blood cholesterol levels. After a meal blood cholesterol levels are misleadingly peaked due to the absorption of digested fats from the food.

Fat in our diet - the good guys and the bad guys

Fats in our diet takes different forms according to its level of saturation- a phenomenon associated with its biochemical structure. This level of saturation cause the particular fat to act differently in increasing or reducing the levels of LDL and HDL cholesterol in our body. Fully saturated or "saturated fat" promotes the generation and deposition of "bad" LDL cholesterol in the body. Less saturated fat called mono and poly unsaturated fats help reduce the levels of LDL cholesterol. It is important to minimize and if possible completely avoid saturated fats. Moderate amounts of mono and poly unsaturated fat is considered beneficial. Animal fat is made of predominantly saturated fat. Therefore beef, chicken, pork and other meat products contain high amounts of saturated fats. Vegetable oils such as olive oil, sunflower oil and canola oil are predominantly made of unsaturated fats. Some vegetable oils too such as coconut oil have large amounts of saturated fats.

Saturated fats

These fats are mainly derived from animal sources. Saturated fats remain in the solid state at room temperature. These fast are considered unhealthy and contributory to the plaque build up in the arteries and the hardening of the arteries. They cause the elevation of the levels of harmful LDL cholesterol and decrease the levels of HDL cholesterol in the blood stream.

Sources of saturated fats (that you should avoid as much as possible)- cocoa butter, palm oil, coconut oil, milk, butter, cheese, beef, pork, eggs, chicken skin, processed meat such as ham, sausage, salami, fried food, baked food and pizza.

Polyunsaturated fats

These fats remain in liquid state at room temperature. Main source of these fats are vegetable oils. Up to 10 percent of total calorie intake each day should be from polyunsaturated fatty acids. These fats are known to lower the levels of LDL, which is the "bad" cholesterol. It is also known to cause small reductions in the levels of HDL, which is the "good" cholesterol. Polyunsaturated fats in our diet should come from liquid vegetable oils to avoid consumption of the undesirable "trans" fatty acids.

Sources of polyunsaturated fats (that should make up 10% of your daily calorie intake)- fish, almonds, mayonnaise, soybean oil, corn oil, sunflower oil, safflower oil, sesame oil

Monounsaturated fats

These fats are mainly derived from vegetable sources. They are found in liquid form at room temperature. Up to 20 percent of the total daily calorie intake should be from monounsaturated fats. These fats too are known to reduce LDL the "bad" cholesterol. However unlike the polyunsaturated fats, these are known not to lower the levels of the "good" HDL cholesterol. But in fact there is evidence to suggest that monounsaturated fats cause the HDL levels to go up.

Sources of monounsaturated fats (that should make up 20% of your daily calorie intake)- chicken, fish, olive oil, grape seed oil, canola oil, peanut butter, cotton seed oil, avocado

Trans fats

Trans fats are a variety of man made fats that have been altered chemically to resemble the properties of saturated fats. The effect of trans fats in your body is much worse than that of saturated fats. Trans fats are known to elevated the levels of "bad" LDL cholesterol and reduce the levels of "good" HDL cholesterol in the blood thus promoting atherosclerosis that clog up your arteries. Hydrogenated fats, partially hydrogenated fats (such as some margarines-*check the labels*) and vegetable shortening contain high amounts of trans fats. Trans fats are abundant in commercially prepared food because it adds to the texture and the taste. Trans fats have preservative properties that help store food for longer periods thus improving their commercial value to the food producers. Even those foods that are labeled as low fat or low in saturated fats may have high amounts of trans fats hidden and unaccounted for. Good way of estimating the level of trans fat is to subtract the total amount of saturated and other forms of fat, as stated in the label, from the total amount of stated fat. This difference is often the amount of trans fat contained in the particular food. Therefore margarines and foods prepared using them such as cakes pastries and biscuits should be avoided or substituted where possible.

Food cholesterol

Although most of the cholesterol found in our bloodstream is manufactured within the body itself dietary consumption of cholesterol too contributes to the elevation of blood cholesterol level. Cholesterol is found only in animal fats. The similar fatty product found in plant sources is called ergosterol. Recommended daily intake of cholesterol is 300mg. Egg yolk is a very rich source of cholesterol. Another rich source of cholesterol is animal liver.

Fish omega-3 fatty acids and heart disease

Fish oil and some plant oils contain beneficial fats in the form of omega 3 fatty acids. Fish oil in fact is given in tablet form to control certain forms of high blood cholesterol levels.

Scientific research has shown that consumption of fish oils and omega 3 fatty acids in fish brings great benefits to the heart. These beneficial effects seem to be due to multiple factors associated with fish oil and omega 3 fatty acids. It has a very beneficial effect on the heart muscle cell by contributing to its proper function. It also has a blood thinning effect that renders protection from heart attacks. Fish oil intake also seems to contribute to blood pressure control. Omega3 fatty acids and fish oil help control blood cholesterol levels. It has been described that fish and fish oil help prevent coronary artery disease as well sudden death due to heart disease.

Fish such as mackerel, lake trout, herring, sardines, albacore tuna and salmon contain high levels of omega-3 fats. The American heart association recommends eating at least two servings of fish per week.

Guidelines for a heart healthy diet-What fat containing food to avoid?

Choose sauces, gravies and dressings that contain low fat content. Avoid heavy cream, butter, full cream milk and products thereof, margarine, mayonnaise or animal fats. Choose lean meats and skinless poultry. Always remove the fat from meats before cooking.

When choosing milk, dairy products and food made of dairy always go for the low-fat or fat-free varieties. Choose the low fat versions of the cheeses. Remember that non-dairy creamers too can contain saturated fats and better be avoided.

Develop the habit of reading the food labels and the nutritional information always. Note the total fat level per serving, the different fats contained and the total calories per serving. Always select the food with lowest total fat content, those with no saturated fats and those with a low total calorie levels. Choose food with no or low fat. Where fat is present select those with high levels of mono or polyunsaturated fatty acids. Avoid or minimize the consumption of foods containing hydrogenated oils that are rich in trans fats. High levels of hydrogenated fats are found also in fries, chips and other fried and baked foods. Consume more seafood and fish.

Avoid frying your food. If necessary, fry only with oils containing monounsaturated fats such as olive oil. It is desirable to broil, grill or bake and avoid frying altogether. Recommended vegetable oils include extra virgin olive oil, safflower oil and canola oil. Avoid butter, lard, tallow and ghee where possible. Avoid palm oil and coconut oil that is rich in saturated fats.

Plant sterol and stanol esters

Plant sterols and stanol esters have been shown to be very effective in helping to reduce the blood cholesterol levels. The cholesterol reduction brought about by these dietary constituents can be up to 10-14%. Recommended amounts for plant sterols is 0.65 grams per day or and for stanol esters it is 1.7 grams per day.

Plant sterols and stanol esters can be obtained from the following foods

Vegetable oil (esp. soy oil), nuts, seeds, cereals, legumes
Spreads and salad dressings (check the label)

Carbohydrates: Good carbohydrates, bad carbohydrates and the glycemic index

Carbohydrates are essential ingredients of your daily diet. It is important to understand the different qualities of different carbohydrate containing foods to appreciate their effect on your body and your health. Carbohydrate containing foods are classified according to a concept called the glycemic index (GI). The carbohydrates we eat get broken down to simple sugars like glucose and fructose for absorption in the intestines. Once absorbed most sugars appear in the blood as glucose. glycemic index gives and idea of how much of an effect each carbohydrate containing food has on the blood glucose level shortly after its consumption. The glycemic index is therefore a ranking of foods based on their immediate effect on your blood glucose level. It measures how much the blood glucose level increases over a period of two or three hours after a meal. Foods that cause the blood sugar level to rise immediately after digestion and absorption are foods with a high glycemic index. Such foods provide high amounts of calories per unit consumed and thus contribute to excess energy that gets converted to fats. Excess consumption of foods with high glycemic index will lead to excess fat synthesis and deposition, weight gain and obesity. Foods with a high glycemic index are particularly bad for the diabetics because it causes the blood sugar levels to go up sharply making proper control of its levels difficult. Excess consumption of such foods can also lead to the early development of diabetes in those who are at risk such as those with a family history of diabetes or those who are over weight. It also contributes to the development of heart disease and stroke by indirect means.

It is recommended that more of the carbohydrates in your diet be from foods with a low glycemic index. When eaten, these foods cause only a slow and low elevation of your blood glucose level. These carbohydrates are broken down slowly releasing glucose gradually into your blood stream. Foods with a low glycemic index help control your appetite and decrease your food cravings (by decreasing the secretion of hormones that stimulate food cravings). These foods generate less energy. So your body may start breaking down fat deposits for energy production. This may lead to weight loss. These foods also make the blood sugar control easier in the diabetics.

The glycemic index of each carbohydrate containing food should be considered the best measure of how good or bad a particular food is for your health. You should avoid foods with a high glycemic index as much as possible.

In the past carbohydrate containing foods were classified according to the complexity of the particular chemical structure of the carbohydrates in it. The relevance of this classification is now questioned. The complexity of the chemical structure has little effect on the glycemic index. Simple carbohydrates such as cane sugar (made of sucrose) cause your blood sugar level to rise very high soon after its consumption. Complex carbohydrates such as rice or potatoes also can cause your blood sugar level to rise sharply, thus they too have a high glycemic index. But basmati rice and brown rice are considered to have a lower glycemic index. Channa dhal has a very low glycemic index. The following table gives you an idea of the different glycemic indexes of different carbohydrate containing foods.

Food with a low glycemic index is recommended for better general health and better cardiac health. You should familiarize your self with the glycemic indices of many common carbohydrate-containing foods. Armed with this knowledge, always remember to choose foods with a low glycemic index.

Low GI carbohydrates desirable in moderation

1. Low fat plain yogurt (14)
2. Cherries (22)
3. Lentils (26)
4. Skim milk (32)
5. Apple (38)
6. Pears (38)
7. Chick pea (42)
8. Orange (44)
9. Peas (48)
10. Carrots (49)
11. Whole meal bread (53)
12. Banana (55)

High GI food that should be avoided or absolutely minimized

1. Steamed white rice (98)
2. Puffed wheat (89)
3. Jacket potato (85)
4. Cornflakes (84)
5. French fries (75)
6. Bagel (72)
7. White bread (70)
8. Mashed potato (70)

Soy

Soy is a very heart healthy food variety. It is known to help reduce your blood cholesterol levels and lower your blood pressure. Processed soy is available in many forms. Nutrition authorities recommend the consumption of 25 grams of soy protein per day. Soy is recommended as a major substitute for animal protein in the diet of those who have high blood cholesterol levels. For such individuals the recommended soy protein intake per day is 25-50 grams.

Soy is considered very protective to the heart. This protective effect may be due to its high content of isoflavones. Isoflavones act in a similar manner to human estrogen that protects women against heart disease prior to menopause. Isoflavones also possess antioxidant properties.

It is important to read the labels of the food products containing soy. Ensure you check the soy protein content as well as the isoflavone content of each product per serving. It is noteworthy that some soy products may have its isoflavones removed during processing. Always remember to choose soy products with high isoflavone content.

Isoflavone levels of different soy products

Food type	Isoflavone content
1. Tempeh (cooked half a cup)	54mg
2. Soybean oil	0mg
3. Silken tofu (slice)	21mg
4. Soy sauce (tablespoon)	2mg
5. Soy floor (cup)	130mg
6. Dry roasted soy bean	150mg

Antioxidants

Harmful chemicals in your blood called super radicals cause damage to the endothelium lining the inner wall of your arteries. Cholesterol plaque deposition happens in areas of the artery wall thus damaged. These super radicals are destructive to your body and they also accelerate your body's aging process. Antioxidants are chemical compounds that can fight and neutralize those harmful super radicals. Thus the intake of antioxidants in our diet or in the form of supplements may help prevent the harmful effects of super radicals and contribute to the prevention of diseases like heart disease.

There have been many reports to suggest that antioxidants such as vitamin C, vitamin A and beta-carotene can lead to the prevention of heart disease and death. Whilst there have been some scientific validity to this notion a very reliable study published recently failed to prove this conclusively. However the theoretical fact remains that harmful super radicals can cause damage to organs and cells in the body contributing to the development of many diseases including heart disease and accelerate the aging process. Such super radicals are kept under control by antioxidants. Fresh vegetables, fruits and tea are rich in antioxidants and the regular consumption of it may bring about health benefits. Value of antioxidant supplements as tablets and formulas has not been definitively proven. But the regular consumption of natural foods with high antioxidant levels is highly recommended.

Mediterranean diet

A study in the 1950s showed that people living in the Greek island of Crete had a very low incidence of heart disease and certain types cancers. They also lived long lives. Researchers later found out that such good health and longevity was enjoyed by not only the people of Crete but also the people living all over Greece and Southern Italy. The reason for this state of good health and longevity was attributed to their dietary patterns. Their traditional diet, believed to be beneficial for good health, gave rise to the concept of the heart healthy Mediterranean diet. The Mediterranean diet consists of large amounts of fruits, vegetables, legumes, whole-grain cereals, nuts, and olive oil. Surprisingly their fat intake was still relatively high. But the fat in their diet was predominantly olive oil, which is rich in mono unsaturated fats. This diet also included moderate amounts of fish and poultry. The red meat content of this diet was very low. They also consumed red wine in moderate amounts regularly with their diet.

A landmark medical study called the Lyon heart study put the Mediterranean diet to scientific test. The results of the study showed that adopting the Mediterranean diet helped people with heart disease fair better. It contributed to the prevention of further heart attacks and also death from heart disease in these people. Mediterranean diet is one of the only two diets that have scientifically been proven to save lives.

Indo- Mediterranean diet

This is another diet that has been proven by scientific research to be beneficial to heart health. This diet too is based on the principles of the Mediterranean diet and consists mainly of plant foods. In addition to the constituents of the Mediterranean diet this diet contains foods consumed in the Indian subcontinent. Heart disease and risk factors for heart disease are observed to be very rare among the villagers in India that predominantly consume the traditional Indian vegetarian diet. This Indo-Mediterranean diet is basically made up of soybean oil, mustard oil, fresh vegetables, fruits, nuts and whole grain. Regular and long-term adoption of this diet has shown to reduce the incidence of heart attacks and sudden death from heart attacks in those who are at a high risk.

Tea and cardiac health

Tea contains high levels of anti oxidant compounds called flavonoids and catechins. These elements are considered to have a protective effect on the heart and the endothelium of the coronary arteries.
Studies carried out in Europe showed that regular consumption of black tea reduced the incidence of heart disease and death from heart disease. Experts agree that tea drinking should be promoted as a healthy dietary habit.

Sodium

Excess consumption of salt (sodium chloride) is known to contribute to high blood pressure. Therefore it is encouraged that those with high blood pressure consume food with no added salt. This is true for patients suffering from heart failure too. Salt intake causes you to drink more water since it stimulates thirst. But those with heart failure have dfficulty removing water from the body. Thus excess intake of water caused by the intake of salt may lead to fluid overload and worsening of body swelling and the swelling of the lungs in these individuals. This leads to worsening of the heart failure symptoms.

It has been observed that an adult consumes around 10grams of salt per day in the US. Recommended daily consumption of salt is less than 2.5 grams per day. So we are a nation of excess salt consumption. It is no wonder that high blood pressure is so prevalent in this country. Most processed foods and fast food contain high salt levels. Foods with high salt content that should be avoided or restricted include chips, crackers, cheese, instant pre-prepared food (noodles, soups, stews), fast food, sausages, ham, salted nuts, smoked meat, smoked fish, soy sauce and pickles.

Homocysteine and Folic acid

Homocysteine is a naturally occurring amino acid in our body, as described earlier. It is generated by the break down of proteins in the diet. It is one of the essential amino acids that the body needs for the building of tissues. While normal levels are desirable, elevated level of homocysteine can lead to heart disease. Homocysteine has a harmful effect on the endothelium lining the blood vessels. Such effects lead to the increased occurrence of cholesterol plaques in the coronary arteries. While accelerating the narrowing of the blood vessels by cholesterol plaques, elevated homocysteine also causes your blood to clot easily. Such blood clots formed within the blood vessels cause heart attacks and strokes.

So elevated homocysteine levels are considered to be a risk factor for heart disease and stroke. It is considered to be one risk factor that causes heart attacks in those who have no other conventional cardiac risk factors. Homocysteine accumulates in your body when it is not broken down adequately. Homocysteine level in your blood should be less than 10 micromoles per liter. Folic acid is an important factor that helps your body to breakdown homocysteine. Vitamins B12 and B6 too are necessary for this breaking down process.

Consumption of adequate levels of folic acid, vitamin B12 and vitamin B6 can lower your risk of suffering heart attacks and strokes. These vitamins benefit primary as well as secondary prevention of heart attacks and strokes. Supplementation of these vitamins also help reduce the re narrowing of coronary arteries after they have been opened by coronary angioplasty and stenting.

Foods that contain high levels of folic acid
Dried beans, Liver, Lentils, Pears, Broccoli, Whole grain, Brussels sprouts, Spinach, Beet root, Oranges

Foods that contain high levels of vitamin B6
Meat, Fish, Milk, Eggs

Food that contain high levels of vitamin B12
Whole grain, Fish, Chicken

Red Wine

There is a peculiarly low incidence of heart disease in France despite their diet being similar to that of the rest of the West. For many years it has been speculated that relatively higher rates of red wine consumption may be the factor behind the relatively better heart health the French enjoy. Recently researchers in the UK have described a compound called polyphenol, present in grape skin and rich in red wine to be very effective in decreasing the production of a harmful protein called endothelin-1 in your body. Endothelin-1 is known to cause blood vessels to shrink and this is one key mechanism by which a heart attack happens. In addition the polyphenols in red wine have anti oxidant properties. Consumption of a glass of red wine each day is considered to be optimal to cardiac health.

Alcohol

Research involving red wine revealed its benefits in the prevention of heart disease. Later these benefits were found out to be relevant not only to red wine but to other forms of alcohol too. However benefits can be obtained only by drinking small amounts alcohol (about 10 grams each day) on a regular basis. It should be cautioned that any excess of that could lead to organ damage and alcohol dependence. Alcohol in excess can elevate blood pressure, cause obesity, lead to liver, pancreas, heart and brain damage and cause psychological ill health.

Practical application of dietary change – "food watching"

As has been described dietary habits have far reaching implications as far as your heart health is concerned. It is often very confusing to analyze your diet to see how much harm it is doing to you. It is even more nerve wrecking to correct and optimize your diet to make it more healthy. This confusion is partly due to the plethora of information that you are bombarded with from many different and diverse sources. Often such information may be conflicting and contradictory thus adding to the confusion. Therefore it is important to learn the simple approaches to analyzing your current diet and find out what changes you have to do to make it healthier.
Healthy eating habits may prevent not only heart disease but also many other disorders including some cancers and even psychological maladies. First step in the journey to healthy eating is acquiring the essential knowledge on the healthy and unhealthy foods. Then you should learn to distinguish the two. When you know what is good and what is bad for you to eat, you have the power of choice. The second step is to acquire motivation and desire to exercise wise dietary choices. The combination of the above two steps will help you completely change the way you look at food and change to the better what you eat. Do not let others feed you "poison". It is your heart and your life, so try to take charge. Eat what is good for your health and for your life –by choice.

Some simple actions can start the process of renewal of your eating habits. You should always remember that from now on you are eating not just to satisfy your taste buds or to respond to your hunger. But you are eating to live healthy and to fill your life with vitality. Think of it also as a cleansing process. By deliberately eating good and healthy food, you are cleaning up the organs and the systems in your body of all the dirty "stains" and "grease" of the bad food you used to eat before.

First make a list of the different foods that you ate with each meal over the last week or two. This should include the main meals as well as any other meals and snacks. Now go through your list and identify the foods that you seem to eat more frequently and underline them with a red pen. Then in the light of what you have learnt form reading this chapter, identify the bad foods – those with high fat content, bad fat combinations, red meat, high glycemic index and high calories etc. Cross these out with a pen. Now against each type of food that has been crossed out write a good type of food that you may have eaten instead. The good foods include fresh fruits, fresh vegetables, fish, nuts, legumes, fibre and whole grain products etc. (remember the Mediterranean and the Indo-Mediterranean diets). Now what you have in your paper is the basic blue print for a new and healthy diet that suits you.

The next step is to eat the good types of food by deliberate choice as often as you can. You should start keeping a log of what you eat each day. Remember to read the nutritional information on the labels of what you eat and note down the estimated amount of calories, fat, fat types and sodium you are consuming. At the end of the week go through your log and see where you may have crossed the line and eaten some thing that is bad. Also try to calculate and estimated the total amount of calories you may have eaten each day. If you have eaten more calories than you are supposed to eat try to figure out how you could cut down on the excess calories each day. Check whether you have eaten more sodium than you are supposed to. Check the total amount of fat you may have eaten each day and amounts of different types of fat. Identify once again the bad foods that you should avoid in the future – those that contain high amounts of sodium, saturated fat, trans fats etc. This practice is called food watching. It is different to regimental dieting. Lessons thus learned should help you to plan better your diet for the next week. Practicing these simple steps for a few weeks will generate within you a habit of eating well and healthy. Choosing healthy food and limiting the portion sizes of the food you eat may become an automatic activity for you. You may thus make a significant change in your life style with minimum effort and disruption to your current life style. By doing this you are embarking on a self initiated process of self-renewal. You make informed choices with reason. It is completely different to reluctantly putting your self through a strict diet planned by some one else. Thus there is a higher chance of you succeeding this way in changing your diet and sticking to it.

As you make these changes to your diet you will start to feel the renewed vitality and energy the healthy diet brings to you. You may also notice weight-loss. Your doctor may see improvements in your blood pressure, blood sugar level and blood cholesterol level. Above all you will realize that you are in charge of your health and your destiny! It is such a good feeling you will love every bit of it – go on try it and experience it for your self!

Practical tips for "food watching"

1. Know than what you eat will decide how healthy you will be
2. Eat three regular meals a day and eat small to medium sized portions to satisfy your appetite
3. Avoid snacks in between meals, particularly those with high fat content (chips, fried food etc.), sweet meats (chocolate, cakes etc.) and processed foods such as cookies etc. If you are still hungry eat fresh fruits or roasted/ non-salted nuts.
4. Avoid non-lean meats, full cream dairy products, candy, chocolate, large amounts of food made of potato, wheat, white rice etc.
5. Read food labels. Develop an appreciation of the calorie values of different foods. Calculate your daily calorie intake and try not to exceed your daily calorie requirements.
6. Cut down on fat (particularly saturated fats, hydrogenated fats, cholesterol)
7. Cut down carbohydrates with high glycemic index
8. Use monounsaturated oils for cooking
9. Eat more fresh vegetables, fruits, nuts (not cooked in oil), legumes and fibre. Use fat free salad dressings
10. Consume a small amount of red wine (one glass per day)
11. Eat more fish, tofu and other soy products and drink more tea
12. Drink plenty of water, drink your one glass of red wine each day

13. Avoid excess salt and high-salt food
14. Keep the food diary and regularly review to see your progress and identify the improvements to be made.

Will low carb-hi protein diets help my health?

Popular low-carb diets advocate drastic reductions in the amount of carbohydrates you consume each day. This forces your body to burn the stored fat to generate energy necessary for your daily activities. We usually eat about 130 grams of carbohydrates each day. Low-carb diets have less than 20 grams of carbohydrate per day. These diets also allow liberal consumption of protein and all types of fat containing food. Due to excessive fat burning people on these diets do lose weight.

Long-term health effects of these diets have not been studied. It has very potent effect in causing you to lose weight fairly quickly. But there also have been reports of various different untoward side effects associated with these diets. Dehydration is one such problem. In the short-term dehydration can cause headaches. But long-term dehydration can have a bad effect on your kidneys. Excessive dehydration can trigger heart attacks too. Due to increase break down of fatty acids there may be a build up of acids in your blood. High acidity will affect the proper balance of different chemicals in your blood leading to abnormalities of your heart rhythm and neurological function.

Low-carb diets lack fibre. The immediate effect of the combination of dehydration and lack of fibre is constipation. In addition lack of fibre in your diet in the long term can lead to many health problems including colon cancer. Deficiency of other nutritional factors such as minerals and vitamins in this diet can potentially cause problems of vision, skin, hair, mouth, and even compromise body immunity.

While this diet is effective in causing weight loss it may not be too good for your heart's health. If you have coronary risk factors or if you are have heart disease it is advisable not to go on a low carb-hi protein diet. Instead heart healthy diet based on the principles of diet watching and calorie watching should be emphasized as the best alternative. These diet plans are based on the Mediterranean and Indo-Mediterranean diets that have proven cardiovascular benefits and life prolonging qualities. In addition these diets advocate gradual restriction of calories, carbohydrates with a high glycemic index and fat. As such these diets too could bring equivalent weight loss while protecting your heart.

Chapter 7

Jump, run and live to the max

Physical exercise offers significant health benefits to people of all ages. These benefits include physical health as well as mental health. Long-term exercise helps in the risk factor modification, primary prevention and secondary prevention of coronary heart disease. Many doctors fail to promote and use physical exercise as a tool for good health in their patients. Regular physical exercise is a good health practice that should be an important part of your daily life style. In that it is an investment of sorts. Exercising for good health is different to competitive sports or adventure sports. You should know some basic facts about the suitable types of exercise that will bring you the anticipated health benefits. The basic questions that you need to answer in this regards include why you should exercise, what kind of exercise is optimal, when to exercise and for how long and how often?

Benefits of physical exercise are immense to those who have suffered heart attacks, those who suffer from angina and those who have other types of heart disease including heart failure. But it should be borne in mind that the healthy as well as those with heart conditions should exercise within clearly stipulated guidelines and under some supervision or guidance of a health care provider to avoid potential harm and injury. It is always important to talk to your doctor prior to embarking on an exercise program. Doctor can assess your level of physical fitness and review your cardiac risk factor profile. Your doctor can give valuable advice on whether it is safe for you to embark on a physical exercise program.

A health check with the doctor prior to starting physical exercise may involve a detailed history and a physical examination. Doctor may recommend an exercise stress test to check whether you have any potential limitations or health risks of exercising. If you have coronary risk factors and you have been relatively inactive for a

while you may have developed blockages in your coronary arteries, but with no symptoms. This can potentially put you at risk of a heart attack if you were to engage in physical exercise that your body is not accustomed to.
The stress test can also assess your level of physical fitness. During this stress test if you were to experience shortness of breath on relatively low exertion or experience any discomfort that may signify possible effort related angina your doctor will refer you to get further tests. These tests may also include a coronary angiogram. Doctor can also estimate your level of physical fitness by monitoring your heart rate and your blood pressure and measuring the duration over which you could exercise at progressively higher levels of intensity. After the health and fitness assessment most doctors will give you recommendations on the types of exercise you could do and the intensity at which it should be performed.

Aerobic exercise

Aerobic exercise is activity performed with the energy generated by burning body fuels (glucose) using oxygen. Continuous low to moderate speed activity or movements utilizing the large muscles of arms and legs are typically aerobic in nature. Walking, jogging, cycling, skiing and dancing are some such exercises. Aerobic exercise makes your heart and lungs work harder to maintain a constant supply of blood and oxygen to the working muscles. Thus it places some demand on your heart. With aerobic activity your heart's pump function (contractility), heart rate and your blood pressure all increase. To maintain a constant and elevated level of oxygen supply, your breathing becomes deeper and faster. Aerobic exercise in fact places great demands on your whole body. Regular aerobic exercise trains your muscles, heart and lungs to work harder and more efficiently. This training improves your level of physical fitness. In addition because of the energy generated, body's energy reserves stored as fat gets burnt. This facilitates weight loss. Regular exercise also lowers your resting blood pressure, blood cholesterol level and blood glucose level. Aerobic exercise should makes up the core component of your exercise program. The potential health benefits of regular aerobic exercise are overwhelmingly high.

Benefits of regular physical exercise

1. Improves the efficiency of heart function and lung function and your general physical fitness

2. Lowers your resting heart rate due to the increased efficiency of heart's pumping function (the heart works with ease)

3. Lowers your blood pressure

4. Facilitates weight loss / prevents obesity

5. Reduces blood cholesterol level

6. Reduces the overall risk of coronary heart disease by risk factor modification as well as by improving heart's working capacity

7. Helps control blood sugar levels

8. Improves body immune system

9. Reduces stroke risk

10. Reduces the risk of certain cancers

11. Improves your sense of well being and adds quality to your life

12. Provides mental relaxation and stress relief

13. Improves balance and coordination

14. Provide relief from anxiety and depression

15. Improves sleep and healthy appetite

Anaerobic threshold

This is a technical term that denotes the amount of work you can perform at very high speed. Such high intensity activity is possible only for very short periods of time. The initial portion of any activity involving the use of large limb muscles happens under anaerobic circumstances. In this phase your muscles utilize the fuel stored within them to generate a short burst of energy. This energy production happens with no oxygen utilization and thus it cannot last for too long. This is due to the limited supply of fuel available in the muscle tissue that can generate energy without oxygen. These high-energy stores are made of chemical compounds called creatinine phosphate (CP) and adenosine tri phosphate (ATP). The initial phase where your muscles act using only the stored energy reserves of CP and ATP is called the anaerobic phase of your exercise. And amount of exercise you can perform without oxygen is your anaerobic threshold.

After you start the activity and the repetitive movement of your large muscles their blood supply surges to very high levels. This blood brings along oxygen that the muscle needs to burn glucose and other fuels to continue on with the activity. This phase in which the energy production is done by burning (oxidizing) fuel with oxygen is called the aerobic phase. As you become more and more physically fit your anaerobic threshold will increase. Increased anaerobic threshold reflects improved cardiovascular health too.

Resistance Training

This term represents the exercise done by performing limb movements against some form of resistance such as free weights, spring-loaded pulleys or a stationary object. Exercise done by exerting pressure against a stationary object (resistance) is called isometric exercise. Scientists advocate incorporation of resistance training to regular exercise programs. Resistance training contributes only minimally to the improvements in cardiovascular or lung fitness. Its main effect is to improve muscular strength. It is also known to contribute significantly to the feeling of well being brought about by exercising.

Benefits of resistance training

1. Improve muscular strength and muscular endurance
2. Improve bone density - thus contributing to the prevention of osteoporosis

Stretching

Stretching of joints and muscles is an integral part of any physical exercise program. It improves joint and muscular flexibility and increases joint range of motion. Stretching should be performed at the beginning of any physical exercise session to prepare muscles for the subsequent increased activity. It is a part of the warm up process. Stretching help increase blood flow to the relevant muscles. It also helps prevent joint and muscular injury. Stretching should be performed at the end of an exercise session too. This is the process of gradual warming down. Warming down also helps prevent muscular injury. Stretching can also prepare tendons and muscles for the upcoming exercise. It is known to help prevent the delayed onset -muscle soreness (DOMS), which is the soreness you experience in the days immediately following a workout. Stretching help mentally prepare you for the workout. Exercise such as yoga predominantly involves stretching.

Remember, safety first

Even if your doctor has given you the all clear it is still important that you adhere to proper guidelines and safety precautions as you exercise. Ensuring adequate hydration, wearing loose and proper clothing and comfortable and safe footwear are important aspects to be mindful of. If you were to experience any discomfort particularly chest tightness, shortness of breath or ache that runs along your neck or left or right arm it is absolutely important that you see your doctor about it before exercising again. It is important to make sure that what you are experiencing is not angina.

Designing a suitable exercise program

The expert authorities such as the American College of Sports Medicine advocate exercising at least 3 to 5 times a week. This may take the form of a brisk walk, jog, run, cycling or even playing a sport. Prior to commencing the aerobic segment, you should spend 5-10 minutes on stretching your arms, legs, neck and the torso (see figure – some stretching movements).
How hard you exercise should be decided on your level of physical fitness. Intensity is defined in terms of your maximum possible heart rate. If you are unfit it is advisable to start the program at an intensity where you reach only 50% of your maximum heart rate at the peak of the exercise session. Your maximum possible heart rate is calculated by subtracting your age from the number 220. An electronic heart rate monitor that can be worn on your wrist may help assess your heart rate while exercising. Some exercise machines have a built in heart rate sensor in the handle. Otherwise you can manually measure it by feeling and calculating the carotid pulse in your neck (located in either side of the neck about an inch below the jaw). As you progress along you can increase the intensity of your activity as you feel comfortable, over time.

You should perform aerobic exercise for at least for 20-40 minutes per session.
As you progress with the aerobic exercise program you may also incorporate some resistance training to the routine. This may take the from of light free weights (in the form of dumbbells or barbells), spring loaded exercise machines or even a heavy object like a big book that can be gripped firmly and safely. You may spend one fourth of your session time on resistance training. Resistance training should be commenced under the supervision of a qualified trainer because of the propensity to injure your self if done improperly.

As you become familiar with resistance training you may be able to isolate the different muscles or the group of muscles you train with each type of movement. It is important that your workout be balanced where both sides of the body are exercised to the same level. Your trainer should guide you on the number of repetition per each set and the number of sets of each exercise type, depending on the relative strength and weakness of each muscle group. Three sets of five repetitions for each type of resistance exercise is a good basic guideline to start with.

You will feel the positive effects of exercise from the first session it self. Increased vitality and feeling of well-being are felt very early. Over time you will notice weight loss and improved body image. Your doctor will notice improvements in your blood pressure, blood cholesterol level and blood sugar level. As exercise becomes a part of your life style you will know that you are in-charge of your health and well-being. This sense of power and responsibility should be your motivation to give physical exercise its due importance.

Chapter 8

The key to the lock- Interventional Cardiology (Pinhole heart surgery)

Cindy was a 27 year old successful Broadway producer enjoying a brilliant career. She loved life. She loved New York and enjoyed its fast phase, the ever-changing colors, the theaters, galleries, restaurants, nigh clubs as well as the outdoors. When I first saw her in my office I was taken aback for a brief moment. She did not fit the prototype of my usual patient. She was slim, tall and vibrant – an epitome of good health. Besides young women in general very rarely suffer heart disease. So her story is rather unique but by no means rare. One week prior to her visit to my office she had been driving down the Brooklyn bridge when she experienced the strange encounter of a black screen descending down the visual field of her left eye. The next moment she lost sight totally in that eye. She found it hard to keep driving and gradually slowed down to the much annoyance of the motorists driving behind her. She could not imagine how she made it to Broadway without an incidence. There she pulled up and stopped the car at the curb some where in Tribeca. She was scared to death. Then she felt her left arm feeling heavy and in the next instance she lost all movement in the left arm and the left leg. Cindy started to panic and cry. She could not move. She could not believe what was happening. After a while seeing no improvement in the weakness Cindy decided to call for medical help. She was taken to the nearest hospital where she was diagnosed with a stroke. Fortunately for her the weakness and the loss of vision in the left eye improved over the next 24 hours. After the agonizing and anxiety filled stay in the stroke unit of the hospital she was transferred to the neurology floor. The doctors treating her did a large number of investigations to ascertain the cause for Cindy's stroke. Cindy had no identifiable risk factor for stroke. She never smoked cigarettes or used illicit drugs, she did not have high blood pressure or even a family history of stroke. Doctors performed multiple tests in a vain effort to identify a cause but failed. Finally they called Cindy's stroke *"cryptogenic"* or due to a hidden cause. However her neurologist knew that a very high percentage of such cryptogenic strokes have been associated with a hole in the heart that facilitate clots to transfer from the veins to arteries un checked. Such clots can find their way into the brain and block an artery supplying blood to the brain causing a stroke. Reports say that young women have such holes in the heart more often than men and older women. They are remnants of a defect that is usually present during the embryonic stage of your development. Usually after birth due to the changes that take place in the directions of blood flow this defect closes off spontaneously. But in about 15% of the population these defect fail to seal off completely. If the defect remains open into adult life it is called a "patent foramen ovale or in short "PFO".

Cindy was referred for a trans-esophageal echocardiogram or a TEE to look for a PFO. In this test you are made to swallow an ultrasound probe that is advanced to the esophagus. Once placed at the appropriate position very close to the heart, the ultrasound probe emits sound waves directed at the heart. It then captures the reflected ultrasound beams from the moving heart and constructs a picture. Lo and behold proving the neurologist's suspicion the TEE showed a substantial PFO in Cindy's heart. The blood in the veins of Cindy's body were mixing up with those of the arteries in the left side of the heart through a small hole in the wall between the right and left atria. In this process, small blood clots that form in the veins where the blood moves slowly instead of getting filtered out in the lungs gets in to the left heart and get sprayed all over the body. If a big enough clot finds its way into an artery that supplies blood to a vital organ like the brain, heart or kidney it can cause damage to that organ. In Cindy's case this happened to be the brain and as a result she suffered a mini stroke. Luckily she recovered fully but many others do not.

Now the main objective of treating Cindy involved preventing her from having another stroke that may perhaps leave her paralyzed permanently –if she were to be unlucky. The treatment options for her included life long blood thinning tablets or a choice between open-heart surgery or pinhole surgery to close the hole in her heart. Due to its convenience, proven safety and efficacy she opted to the latter. Pinhole surgery involves a cardiac intervention where a device is delivered to the heart via a catheter by accessing a large vein in the leg through a needle puncture. We do this procedure under local anesthesia and mild sedation. The patient undergoing this procedure remains practically awake all through the procedure, which usually takes about half an hour to perform.

A week later I operated on Cindy. A catheter was introduced into the large vein in her groin through a needle stick. The small disc like device, which is used to close the hole in Cindy's heart was advanced to the right side of her heart along the catheter. I then precisely and securely placed the device patching the hole between the two upper chambers of her heart while watching it through fluoroscopy (x-ray) and TEE. The procedure was successful and she experienced only minimal discomfort. Once I was satisfied that the device was precisely and securely positioned in the heart closing the hole I removed the catheters from her body.
Cindy was kept overnight at the hospital. She made a rapid recovery and was discharged home the next day. She is back to her normal life once again savoring all the excitement the city of New York has to offer to a healthy young girl. I saw her once more in my office to make sure she was doing well. She indeed was well and talked to me of an exciting new production she was involved with. The twinkle in her eye was enough evidence to tell me how excited and thrilled she was.

Cindy's story highlights the convenience with which doctors address major heart problems using catheter based interventional cardiology techniques. Interventional cardiology is the latest advancement in cardiac care. The technology has improved extremely rapidly to highly sophisticated levels that many heart problems that necessitated open heart surgery can now be performed through needle holes that allow doctors access to blood vessels. The story of how some pioneering doctors made epoch making discoveries that changed the way heart disease is treated is a fascinating one. No account of interventional cardiac treatment is complete without a brief mention of this interesting historical narrative.

A brief history of interventional cardiology

The first catheters used in medicine were long hollow tubes that were used to drain the urinary bladder. The earliest records on the use of catheters date far back to the times of the ancient Egyptian civilization. Accessing the hearts of animals via catheters began fairly recently. The earliest records of catheters being inserted into the heart can be traced back to the 18th century. Hales a French scientist catheterized the heart of a horse using metal pipes and the windpipe of a goose in the early 18th century. It was the French physiologist Bernard that coined the term "cardiac catheterization" in the 19th century to define the use of hollow tubes to access animal hearts. However in humans catheters were still used only for the purpose of draining the urinary bladder up until the early 20th century.

In 1929 a Young German doctor by the name of Werner Forssmann imagined the possibilities of accessing the hearts of live and awake humans using catheters. However his ideas were not welcomed by his colleagues and superiors. But his enthusiasm was so intense that he decided to try inserting a sterile urinary catheter into his own heart through an opening made into the vein in his forearm at the elbow. He inserted the catheter himself and ran to the x-ray department of the hospital to check where the inside end of the catheter ended up within his body. To his great joy the catheter tip was in the right side of his heart as he could see by x-ray. With this crude experiment the era of human cardiac catheterization dawned.

In 1941 two scientists named Cournand and Richards measured heart's pump function using a catheter inserted to the heart. This was the fist time cardiac catheterization was used for medical diagnostic purposes in humans. For their remarkable and revolutionary breakthrough in the discovery of the technique and the use of cardiac catheterization in the diagnostics and therapeutics of cardiology, the Nobel prize for medicine was jointly awarded to Forssmann, Cournand and Richards. At his Nobel reception speech Cournand proclaimed "we have found the key to the lock" referring to cardiac catheterization. Indeed this was the first door to be open and many more followed soon after.

In spite of the wide spread use of the catheterization to study different aspects of heart's anatomy of function, doctors feared to catheterize the coronary arteries. The belief at that time was that engagement and the injection of x-ray contrast into the coronary artery with a catheter would cause cardiac arrest with dire consequences. In 1958 a radiologist at the Cleveland clinic by the name of Dr Mason Sones was studying a defective heart valve with the help of a catheter inserted to the aorta, the big artery just outside of the heart. As he was completing the study the catheter accidentally found its way into the right coronary artery, and incidentally and inadvertently some x-ray contrast material was injected to the coronary artery. While Dr Sones could visualize the coronary artery the patient tolerated the incident unexpectedly very well. So Dr Sones' famous and remarkable accident showed to the medical community and the world that coronary arteries could be engaged safely with catheters and dye or contrast material injected without causing any harm. This opened the way to study the anatomy of the coronary artery as never before in the live human beings.

Soon this technology developed and spread all around the world. Today coronary angiography is one of the most indispensable and commonly performed diagnostic procedures world-over. The technique introduced by Sones was of tremendous use. However his technique was rather complex and involved making a surgical incision in the inner aspect of the elbow to locate the main artery supplying the forearm. The artery thus located was accessed with the catheter, which then was advanced to the heart to engage the coronary arteries.

In 1967 Dr Judkins a pioneering genius refined the Coronary artery catheterization technique introduced by Sones by demonstrating the feasibility of introducing the catheters via the femoral artery (one of the arteries supplying blood to the leg) by making a needle puncture in the groin. His technique did not necessitate making surgical incisions thus was technically very easy and convenient. Judkins' new technique gathered momentum and became popular quickly. Today by far the majority of coronary catheterizations are done though the groin.

Till about 1964 cardiac catheterization was essentially used only to image the coronary arteries. In 1964 Dr Charles T Dotter introduced the concept and the technique of opening narrowed blood vessels by sequentially passing gradually enlarging probes into the vessel. This was called *angioplasty or "dottering".* This technique was the forerunner of the modern day balloon angioplasty of the coronary arteries. A brilliant young Swiss cardiologist by the name of Andreas Gruentzig conceived the idea of attaching a deflated balloon to the tip of a catheter and introducing it to a blocked artery and opening the artery by inflating the balloon. In 1974 he proved to the world that his technique is practical by opening a blocked artery in a human being who was undergoing open-heart surgery. However this technique was not used to open blocked or narrowed coronary arteries till 1977. In 1977 Andreas Gruentzig, after much research work carried out in pig heart models, used balloon angioplasty via a catheter to open a blocked coronary artery in a human being.

Soon this new technology became very popular all over the world. Treatment of narrowed and blocked coronary arteries with angioplasty became one of the main methods of treatment of angina and heart attacks. The technique and the equipments used fast became more and more advanced and refined. However almost 50% of the coronary arteries opened with balloon angioplasty ended up narrowing and blocking up once again after a period of about six months. This compromised the effectiveness and efficiency of balloon angioplasty as a method of treatment for angina and heart attacks. It caused the patients to undergo repeated procedures to reopen those repeatedly blocked arteries. Some patients were eventually referred to by pass surgery. However angioplasty was being performed everywhere. It was a very popular way of treatment. Due to its convenience and popularity angioplasty technology created a multi-billion dollar international industry. Doctors and bio-medical engineers diligently continued research into the ways of improving the quality and efficacy of angioplasty treatment. This research was particularly focused on preventing or reducing the tendency of the once opened arteries to re narrow.

In 1977 doctors introduced the means of placing a slotted metal coil in the segments of the coronary arteries opened by balloon angioplasty. This coil or the "stent" too was introduced to the artery by mounting it on a balloon attached to a catheter. With the use of stents rates of re narrowing or re-blocking of opened coronary arteries could be brought down to about 30% after six months. This enhanced the efficacy of balloon angioplasty as a method of treatment for coronary artery disease. Stents could repair any damage that was to happen to the artery during balloon angioplasty alone. Before the advent of stents such damage to an artery would have meant urgent by pass surgery to the unfortunate patient.

Even with the use of stents still there was a recognizable number of patients that experienced angina or developed heart attacks due to the re narrowing or blocking off of reopened artery. Coronary arteries block off due to the deposition of cholesterol plaques in the inner wall of the artery. But the narrowing within a stent happens due to a different mechanism. Stents block off due to scar formation in the stented segment of the artery. These scars are similar to wound scars you get when you bruise your skin. When the artery is opened with a balloon, the inner surface of the artery is inevitably bruised. So when the stent is placed, a scar is formed over it. In some people this scar formation happen more aggressively than in others. So the proportion of patients that form scar tissue more than what is anticipated experience re narrowing of the artery in the stented segment after about four months.

Doctors could identify certain risk factors that increased the tendency to cause narrowing within a stent. People who had very long blocked segments, those who had small and narrow arteries and those who were diabetic had a higher rate of stent re narrowing or blocking off. But some developed narrowing within the stent even with no risk factor being present. Stent re narrowing necessitating repeat intervention was the Achilles' heel of interventional treatment of coronary artery disease. Much scientific work has been carried out in the past decade to address this vexing problem that caused many patients to suffer from recurrent symptoms of heart disease requiring repeated interventional treatment or referral to by pass surgery. It also was a significant burden on the healthcare budget.

In the late eighties scientists and doctors made a breakthrough in the treatment and prevention of narrowing of the artery within a stent. The first method to show promise in reducing re-narrowing of stented segments of an artery was intracoronary radiation therapy or *brachytherapy*. This method was essentially used to treat those patients who presented with the re-narrowing of a previously stented segment of an artery. Though this technique was very effective there were still patient presenting with repeated narrowing of the stented segments of the coronary arteries. In brachytherapy, doctors introduce a very slim radioactive rod via a catheter into the stented segment of the coronary artery after it has been opened by a balloon-catheter. Instead of ballooning doctors can also open the blocked segment of the artery by shaving off the build up within the stent or by burring through it. The radiation in brachytherapy caused the scar tissue forming cells in the stented segment to die and thus prevented further formation of scar.

In the last two to three years scientists and doctors developed a method to prevent re-narrowing within the stent due to scar tissue formation. They experimented with the drugs used to stop the growth or kill cancer cells and drugs that are used to stop cells from attacking grafted organs like kidneys in the body. They showed that when they coated the stents that were placed in coronary arteries with anti cancer or anti rejection drugs in non-harmful doses it essentially prevented scar formation and re narrowing of the stented segments of the coronary arteries. These they called "coated stents" or drug eluting stents. Major studies done in animal models proved the safety and efficacy of drug eluting stents. These led to the large human trials that were carried out in many large hospitals in the US, Europe and Asia where comparisons were made between the new drug eluting stents and the traditional non-drug coated stents. These multi center trials were carried out according to stringent scientific criteria with random allocation of new drug eluting stents and traditional non-drug coated stents (now also called bare metal stents) in a blinded fashion. Blinding meant that neither the doctor nor the patient knew what type of a stent the patient received during the study. Only the research scientist could trace by serial numbers allocated to the patient, as to who received what type of stent during the follow up period.

These studies revealed beyond any doubt that drug eluting stents were extremely efficacious in reducing and preventing re narrowing of coronary arteries treated with stents. Treatment with drug-eluting stents has become the state of the art in the treatment of blocked coronary arteries. Reduction in the rates of re-narrowing and re-blocking of opened coronary arteries meant that the treatment was permanent in most patients. The number of patients experiencing recurrent symptoms dropped dramatically. Thus the numbers of patients requiring re intervention or referral for by pass surgery too dropped in very significant numbers. Patients with long narrowed segments, those with small arteries and those who were diabetic, that had a higher propensity to re narrow too were responding extremely well to drug eluting stents and their rates of re narrowing too were dramatically decreased.

Many patients that would otherwise have been referred to coronary artery by pass surgery can now be treated with balloon angioplasty and stenting with significant ease and convenience by interventional means ensuring good long term results. Patients with significant and severe coronary artery disease could be treated with a single needle stick and an over night stay in the hospital instead of having the chest opened up and close to a week's stay in hospital as it was with by pass surgery. Some centers with a good safety record and efficient means of follow up of patients even discharge their patients on the same day upon a few hours of observation after treatment with stents. Many patients get back to their normal daily routines and activities within the matter of a day or two after the procedure, unlike after by pass surgery where the full recovery would take weeks and even months in some cases. Drug eluting stents have revolutionized the way coronary artery disease is treated.

Today coronary angioplasty and steting is the most commonly performed interventional treatment all over the world. Many millions of angioplasties are performed every year and the numbers seem to grow exponentially.

Coronary angiography and angioplasty

Treatment of blocked arteries with balloon angioplasty with subsequent placement of a stent is the standard method of treatment for coronary artery disease today. By far the majority of the patients can be treated this way very effectively and safely. The decision on how best the disease of a particular patient is treated is made by the cardiologist. This decision is based upon reviewing the coronary angiogram and taking into account the whole clinical picture of the patient. The factors of important consideration include the severity of the disease, heart functional capacity (how much of the hearts function is preserved), age, other health problems, the symptoms of the patient and importantly the expectations and the goals of the patient and the family. Some patients with diffuse and severe disease affecting all three arteries of the heart may best be treated with by pass surgery. The same applies to those with disease of the main artery supplying the left side of the heart. However such patients too are treated with balloon angioplasty and stents in increasing frequency nowadays. As technology improves, this trend will further increase.

The process of coronary catheterization involves the patient admitting to the hospital. Patient should have fasted for a period of four to six hours. An empty stomach is important to keep the patient ready in case emergency surgery was to be required. It also prevents patients becoming nauseous and vomiting during the procedure. During the procedure the doctor accesses a big artery of the patient's groin, elbow or wrist by needle puncture under local anesthesia. On most occasions patient remains widely awake or mildly sedated during the procedure. Upon accessing the artery, doctor passes the long, narrow and hollow tubes called catheters in to the heart arteries through gentle manipulation. Once the artery is engaged, a dye, which is an x-ray contrast substance, is injected to the artery while photographing it with an x-ray camera. This part of the process where pictures of the arteries are taken is called coronary angiography. In most straight-forward cases coronary angiography should not take more than ten to fifteen minutes to perform. Once the angiogram is done doctors review it to plan the best strategy of treatment if treatment is required. Doctors may decide to treat the blockades, if there are any, on the same occasion or on a later date according to the individual situation. Some may not need interventional treatment and others may best be treated with by pass surgery. Those who do not require further treatment after an angiogram on the same day can be discharged home in about four hours after the procedure.

Millions of angiograms and angioplasties of the coronary arteries are performed each year. It has established it self as a very safe procedure with minimal complications to the patient. The safety of the procedure is dependent on some important factors such as the competence and the experience of the operator (the doctor), the competence of the center or the hospital, the equipment used and the general health of the patient at the time of the procedure. Doctors who perform these operations a lot are more competent than those who perform lower numbers according to scientific research carried out into the safety of the procedure. Also the centers where many such procedures are performed are considered safer because of their experience and preparedness to address any adverse event. The contemporary equipment with its technical refinement makes the procedure even safer. However as with anything in this world it is not 100% free of complications. In general there is a less than 1% chance of a heart attack, a stroke or death during or as a result of the procedure. Other risks involve bleeding and damage to the arteries that are accessed during the procedure. If any damage were to happen to the coronary arteries during the procedure, on most occasions it can be repaired in the catheterization laboratory itself without causing any inconvenience to the patient. But however on the very rare occasion a patient may require urgent coronary artery by pass surgery.

A patient should tell the doctor of all experience of drug allergy in the past. Allergy to seafood and Iodine too is of importance. This is due to the fact that a history of such allergies may indicate a higher risk of a reaction to contrast dye that is used to inject into the coronary arteries during the procedure. Most often an allergic reaction shows up as an itchy rash or hives soon after the dye is injected. On rare occasions some get a severe form of an allergic reaction called "anaphylaxis" that can even be life threatening. But if known prior to the procedure the patient can very effectively be pre treated with drugs to prevent such allergic reactions.

Stents

Stents are slotted short metal tubes or coils that are inserted to the arteries opened by balloon angioplasty. They in general look like the small spring coils used in self-retractable ball-point pens. Stents acting as scaffolding help to keep the artery from closing once it has been opened with balloon angioplasty. As stated before, stents by them selves cannot prevent re-narrowing of the opened segment of the artery altogether. But the stents coated with drugs that prevent scar tissue formation over the stented segment can prevent narrowing within the stent very effectively.

Prior to the delivery into the body the stent is present in compressed form over a miniature balloon that is attached to the edge of a fine catheter. It is advanced into the coronary artery along a very fine wire. Once placed precisely over the blocked segment of the artery, the balloon is inflated causing the stent to open up. This process in called "stent deployment" Once deployed, the stent stays within the while the balloon is retracted and removed from the body.

Stents are usually made of stainless steel or metal alloys. Most patients do not feel the presence of these small metal structures in their body. Some may experience some chest discomfort no sooner the stent is deployed in the coronary artery. This is considered to be due to the stent stretching the wall of the artery. On most occasions these stents do not set off metal detectors at security check points. Most stents are MRI safe too, however it is important to check with your doctor prior to undergoing MRI scanning.

Comparison with surgery

On the majority of occasions the diseased coronary arteries are amenable to treatment with angioplasty and stents. Early studies done in the era before the discovery of stents showed that patients with a single blocked or narrowed coronary artery or two narrowed arteries benefited more from angioplasty compared to by-pass surgery. However with the advent and the advancement of stent technology these arguments were found out dated and irrelevant. Stenting of the artery after balloon angioplasty was feasible in many coronary arteries and was proven safe and efficacious as much as by pass surgery. The only caveat was that there was a tendency in a minority of patients to experience re-narrowing in the arteries treated with stenting due to scar tissue formation within the stent. Therefore these patients had to undergo repeat procedures. But overall the disease free survival was equal in both groups of patient that underwent by-pass surgery or coronary intervention (angioplasty and stenting). A rough guideline was establish where it is believed that those who had narrowing of multiple coronary arteries with preserved pump function of the heart did very well with catheterization and intervention while those with reduced heart function and very unwell did better with by-pass surgery.

But with the advent of different types of drug coated or drug eluting stents these guidelines will soon have to be changed. With very low proclivity to re-narrow, drug coated stents seem to offer a near permanent outcome to the unblocking of coronaries by angioplasty and stenting. Even the patients with narrowing of the main artery of the left and those with diabetes that performed better with by pass surgery in the past did very well after undergoing angioplasty followed by treatment with drug coated stents. Thus soon the recommendations will have to be changed to treat all kinds of coronary narrowing with drug-coated stents if there are no other contraindications.

Atherectomy and LASER

On the rate occasion, the doctor may find it impossible to open a blocked artery with balloon angioplasty. Without opening narrowed artery stents cannot be deployed. If the plaque blocking the artery has lots of calcium or scar (fibrous) tissue in it, the blockage may be resistant to opening up by balloon angioplasty. Such recalcitrant blocks can be opened by a process called "atherectomy" that involves the mechanical removal of the atherosclerotic plaque. In this process the plaque is literally shaved off and removed. In the late eighties and the early nineties these methods were used widely together with coronary angioplasty. But with the advent of stent technology and its technical advancements atherectomy lost its need for wide usage. So today it is used to open up the more recalcitrant blocks only.

Two commonly used atherectomy methods are called 1. directional atherectomy and 2. rotational atherectomy. The former involves shaving off the cholesterol plaque and the latter involves burring through it. The third method involved opening the artery using LASER beams. LASER atherectomy too was an effective means of opening blocked arteries however it fell out of favor due to its high operational costs and low safety margin. Since of late new more technologically advanced LASER methods are being tested for possible use.

Other heart problems treated with interventions

Many cardiac problems that required open-heart surgery can now be treated safely and effectively through interventional means. So instead of having the chest cut open, most patients can now get their heart problem addressed with a mere needle stick in the groin area. Next to coronary disease the most common need for cardiac surgery was for the repair or replacement of defective heart valves. When valves are diseased they either fail to open adequately to allow the normal passage of blood or they become leaky thus preventing adequate forward flow of blood. On both occasions the valve defect over burdens the heart leading to symptoms and at times -if severe enough- even to death.

Defective valves need either repair or replacement. All valve problems are first studied by the doctors using echocardiographic means of imaging of the heart. Once the anatomical nature of the valve defect is identified, doctors study how the valve defect affects the fluid dynamics or the flow of blood through it. In addition how it has affected the heart's normal function is assessed. The latter functional assessment involves both echo imaging of the heart as well as insertion of catheters in to the heart cavities to record pressure differences across the defective valves. Once such detail is obtained the doctor can decide whether the valve defect could be treated by interventional means or whether it requires surgery.

Interventional cardiologists open narrowed heart valves by passing a precisely sized balloon into the valve opening via an access made in the groin upon needle puncture. The balloon is meticulously placed across the narrowed valve and is inflated in a controlled manner thus reopening the narrowing. This process is called balloon valvuloplasty and has been practiced widely for a fairly long period now.

Doctors have been able to repair or replace altogether, leaky valves by means of interventional techniques. One method of repairing leaky valves involve placing staples or micro sutures in the leaking segment using catheters inserted to the heart through the groin.

Other techniques involve delivery and deployment of balloon mounted heart valves again through an opening in the groin.

Closing holes in the heart

Holes in the heart or septal defects are abnormal communications that persist between the different chambers of the heart. If there is a "hole" or a communication between the two atria it called an atrial septal defect and likewise one between the two ventricles is called a ventricular septal defect. Another form of communication that can exist between the two atria is what is called a patent foramen ovale. Atrial septal defects, patent foramen ovale and ventricular septal defects are usually closed off while the heart is formed in the embryo. Due to largely unknown reasons if these communications fail to close off prior to birth they persist as defects. Some may live with small such defect without any health problems all through their lives. Some such defects that present at birth gradually close off as the person get older. Ventricular septal defects can also be caused by damage done by a large heart attack. But if such defects are big enough to cause large amounts of blood to shunt across heart chambers causing symptoms and heart failure, they need treatment by closure. Patent foramen ovale usually is not big enough to cause shunting of significant amounts of blood. But however it can let blood clots that form in the veins draining the right side of the heart to cross over to the left side. If these small blood clots find their way to the brain and block off an artery this can lead to stroke. Any such symptom or complication associated with holes between heart chambers need treatment. The traditional way of treating such defects involved open-heart surgery. But with the advent of interventional techniques these defects can be treated without having to have the chest opened up for open heat surgery.

Doctors can deliver a device that has the shape of a stud along a catheter that is inserted into the right side of the heart via a needle puncture of the groin. The device then is deployed straddling the defect and sealing the same. Once deployed a natural cell covering forms over the sealing device integrating into the heart's structure. Closure of atrial septal defects and patent foramina ovale is performed very commonly all over the world. Closure of ventricular septal defects is performed in some specialized centers with exceptional expertise. The technology is evolving so fast that it may be available widely in the near future.

Once a device is placed to seal a heart defect the patient is recommended to take aspirin tablets indefinitely. Another medication named clopedigrel too is advised to be taken for the first few months after deployment of the device.

Intravascular ultrasound (IVUS)

Intravascular ultrasound is a miniature ultrasound probe attached to a tip of a catheter that can be introduced into the coronary arteries to obtain ultrasound images of the interior of the artery. The images thus obtained by the ultrasound probe are processed by a computer. Such processed images depict the interior of the artery with great clarity helping the doctors to analyze the anatomy of the blockages to plan the interventional treatment. Intravascular ultrasound also helps the interventional cardiologist to assess the arteries upon treatment with coronary angioplasty and stenting. It helps to assess how effective the treatment to open the blocked artery has been. It also helps the doctor to follow up the treated arteries over time.

Intracardiac echocardiography (ICE)

A small ultrasound probe that acts like a camera can be introduced into the chambers of the heart to take pictures of the inside of these cavities. This too once again is introduced to a blood vessel through a needle puncture in the groin or in the arm and carried to the heart. Once within the heart it takes ultrasound pictures of the inside of the heart. These ultrasound pictures help doctors to study anatomical abnormalities inside of the heart in detail. Thus some forms of heart disorders can be well studied and understood by this means. Subsequently doctors can plan their treatment strategy and once the treatment plan is decided upon, it can be carried out under intracardiac ultrasound guidance. This wonderful technology has been widely used in the treatment of anatomical defects in the heart by interventional means. Intracardiac ultrasound help in carrying out the operation and also in the assessment of the final result.

Renals, carotids

Technology of opening blocked coronary arteries has opened the doors of unlimited possibilities of opening up blocked and narrowed arteries elsewhere in the body too. Most other arteries in the body are larger than the coronary arteries that are not bigger than few millimeters in diameter. So techniques and equipment have been developed to open other relatively bigger arteries elsewhere in the body utilizing the same principles that were utilized to operate on coronary arteries by interventional means – by passing catheters through needle punctures made in the periphery of the body.

Narrowing of the arteries supplying blood to the kidneys can lead to high blood pressure that is usually not very well controlled by blood pressure controlling medications. Some times such narrowing of the arteries lead to decreased kidney function or recurrent swelling of the lungs leading to breathing difficulties.

Narrowing in the arteries that supply the brain can cause strokes. This too happen in a similar manner to heart attacks. Scientific research has shown that opening the narrowings that occur in the neck arteries can help prevent recurrent strikes.

Narrowing of the arteries supplying blood to the leas is a restively common disorder on our society. Patients experience leg pain particularly in the calf area upon walking initially. This pain improves on resting for a moment. This symptom is called "intermittent claudication" in medical jargon. The legend says that Roman emperor Claudius had disease of the leg arteries that made him break his journey regularly when he walked. Thus the name "caludication". Progression of the buildup blockages in these arteries can lead to agonizing pain in the legs at rest and when blood supply is critically reduced even to the formation of non-healing ulcers and death of parts of the feet. Such dying of toes or other areas of feet in called *ischemic gangrene.*

Treatment to all above disorders due to the narrowing of arteries is un blocking of the involved arteries. Traditionally these blocked arteries were opened by performing surgical operations that were often complex and relatively high-risk. Where unblocking is not possible as in the case with advanced arterial disease of the legs, by pass of blocked arteries can be done by surgery. In the extreme cases involved segment of the leg has to be amputated.

But with the advancements made in interventional technology most blocked arteries in the kidneys, neck and the legs can now be opened by interventional means by accessing the arteries through a needle puncture. Patients have found such treatment to be very convenient and preferable to undergoing surgery.

Chapter 9

The way of the woman's heart – Women and heart disease

Simone a 43 year old secretary has been feeling sick for almost three days before she eventually decided see a doctor. She was otherwise well. She smoked half a pack of cigarettes a day. She was not over weight. She tried to eat healthy but never got an opportunity to do any physical exercise. She had to work to meet family's ends and once back at home she had to attend to the household chores.

It all started as a stomachache. She first developed an unusual discomfort in her upper abdomen, just near where the stomach is located. It persisted without abating for a whole day and then she developed nausea and vomiting. She thought her symptoms were caused by the pizza she had for lunch the previous day at work. She found some relief of her discomfort by popping in some antacid tablets that she had in the drug cupboard at home. However by the third day of symptoms she felt quite unwell. She had lost her appetite. She could not keep any food or drink down. So finally she found her way to the family doctor. The doctor examined Simone and thought that she had gastroenteritis. However he was worried that she was very dehydrated. Therefore he recommended admission to hospital for re hydration with an intravenous saline drip. So she ended up in the family medicine floor at hospital for an overnight saline drip. The next day Simone was feeling worse. Her stomach pain has become much severe and she had a mild fever. Doctors started suspecting hepatitis. She was then referred to the gastroeneterologist for further evaluation.

Gastroeneterologist doubted that her symptoms were due to hepatitis. Though the blood tests showed some abnormalities in the liver function it was not bad enough to support a diagnosis of hepatitis. Besides other tests for hepatitis came back negative. She was transferred to the gastroenterology floor subsequently for further evaluation of her "mystery illness". On the fifth day Simone's condition became critical. Her blood pressure dropped and heart rate increased to over hundred beats per minute. She was having terrible breathing difficulties. She was urgently transferred to the intensive care unit. More blood tests were done in the intensive care unit and the doctors noticed that there was evidence of damage to her heart muscle. Her blood troponine levels were extremely high suggesting the possibility of a massive heart attack. Troponine level in blood goes up when some damage happens to the heart muscle. At this juncture I was called in to assess Simone.

When I first saw Simone she was on life support. She was intubated and kept alive by a ventilator. When I studied her EKG I realized that she had suffered a massive heart attack possibly four to five days earlier. I went on to examine her heart function through echo imaging. The front wall of her heart was barely moving due the damage done by the heart attack. The chest x-ray showed fluid collecting in her lungs. Her heart was failing and not pumping enough blood forward. Build up of fluid in the liver was causing some degree of liver damage too. Additionally due to the inadequate blood flow, her kidneys were beginning to fail. Simone's life was in danger. The missed heart attack has caused enormous damage to her heart that there was very little possibility of salvaging her heart muscle. However I decided to perform urgent cardiac catheterization on her to study her coronary arteries and if I could, to unblock the artery that caused the heart attack.

Coronary angiography showed total blockade of the large artery supplying blood to the front wall of her heart. The pump function of her heart had gone down to one third of its normal level. In other words she was in severe heart failure. I went on to open the blocked artery. Usually opening a totally blocked coronary could be challenging and the material clogging up the artery does not give way easily. However I could open Simone's coronary without much difficulty. This ease at which the artery opened suggested to me that it has been blocked very recently. With the blood supply to the affected area of the heart restored Simone made some recovery over the next few days. Her condition improved very slowly. After almost three weeks at hospital Simone was discharged home. I strongly recommended that she continue to attend the cardiac rehabilitation facility in the hospital. Rehabilitation was essential in her case to restore her functional capacity as much as possible and to prevent a repeat heart attack.

Despite my emphatic instructions she failed to come back for rehabilitation. She failed to keep her appointments to see me for follow up. I was hoping that she would be seeing another doctor at her convenience. However I had suspicions that she may not be seeing any doctor at all. My suspicions were proven correct when I saw Simone once again in the ER three months later with another heart attack. This time she was very unwell. Her family told me that she had been practically house bound since the previous heart attack. She has not complied with the tablets I prescribed to her. It was close to midnight on a Saturday. I decided to perform an urgent cardiac catheterization to hopefully open the blocked artery that was causing her heart attack. This would give her the best chance of recovery or even survival. But nature had other plans. Though we were ready to start the operation in no time Simone never made it to the catheterization laboratory. On her way to the lab she had a cardiac arrest. She could not be resuscitated. Simone fell victim to a heart attack at the age of forty three. The only cardiac risk factors she had were physical inactivity and smoking. Simone's story highlights many unique aspects of women and heart disease.

Women and the heart

Nearly half a million women in America die of cardiovascular disease each year. That means one in every three women will die of heart disease. Many hundreds and thousands are affected by cardiovascular disease. Many millions of women are at risk of getting the disease. Since the year 1984 many more women have died of heart disease than men in the US. This gap seems to be ever widening. Many reasons have been identified as causative of this situation. However women's lack of awareness of their own risk has been one main reason in this regard. Taking into consideration the gravity of the situation The American College of Cardiology, American Heart Association and the National Heart, Lung and Blood institute have joined hands in a powerful campaign to raise awareness of heart disease among women.

Many women fear dying of cancer than of heart disease. However mortality from heart disease among women is about five times higher than that from breast cancer. More women know about the dangers of breast cancer than heart disease due to the increased awareness created by public health campaigns on breast cancer. Surveys have revealed that even some doctors are unaware of the comparatively higher mortality associated with heart disease among women. Statistics say that mortality from cancer is lower than from cardiovascular disease. Eight times more women die of heart disease than from breast cancer. Ignorance of the community has led to the development of this situation.

Women and risk of heart disease

Traditionally coronary heart disease was thought to be essentially a disease of men. Therefore all attention at prevention and treatment was centered on men. Even the majority of scientific work carried out into heart disease has been male focused. This exclusive focus has brought about some control in the impact of heart disease on men. But the relative ignorance of its impact on women has led to its increased and growing prevalence among women.

Most scientific research on treatment methods and drugs for heart disease has been conducted on men. There have been many questions raised as to whether the results of such "men oriented" research findings could be applied to the treatment of women too. Current assumption in the medical fraternity is that it does apply to both sexes so therefore common treatment protocols are usually made for both sexes. However more and more research is carried out with women in focus and the incipient major studies try to enroll equal numbers from both sexes.

Coronary heart disease in women has some important and fundamental differences compared to that of men. Women present with heart disease on the average 20 years later than men. This is due to the fact that women are protected from heart disease in the years prior to menopause by the high levels of female hormone estrogen in the circulation. Estrogen, in addition to offering protection from heart disease helps in controlling blood cholesterol levels. However after menopause incidence of heart disease in women increase sharply and by the seventh decade the relative incidence of heart disease become similar in men and women. Interestingly recent observations have identified a trend towards women developing heart disease at much younger years.

With advancements made in the methods of treatment and prevention of heart disease, the mortality form heart disease among men has gone down significantly over the last two decades. However a similar reduction in mortality has not been observed among women. The reason for this is not limited to the physiological difference between the two sexes. It has a sociological aspect too in that less women seek treatment for heart disease and even those who present for treatment present too late. The root cause for this situation is the relative lack of awareness among women on issues of heart health and heart disease. The misnomer that heart disease is a health concern of men only is another factor contributing to this trend. In the global setting the disparity of resources available for men and women for heart disease management may be another contributing factor.

Just as there are fundamental differences in the way heart disease develops and presents between men and women, there are important differences in the way of treatment and treatment outcomes too.

There is evidence to confirm that the benefits of aspirin therapy are equal in both sexes. But the benefits of the all-important cholesterol lowering statin therapy to the woman is still questioned. However, there is emerging evidence to the beneficial effects of aggressive cholesterol lowering with statin drugs among women. There are other conditions that are women specific such as metabolic syndrome associated with obesity, diabetes and polycystic ovaries. This condition predisposes you to developing heart disease. Women with polycystic ovary syndrome and insulin resistance benefit from the treatment with anti-diabetic drugs such as metformin (Glucophage) and rosiglitazone (Avandia).

There are some differences noticed in the way men and women are treated by interventional means. In comparison to men women who get treatment for heart disease by balloon angioplasty and stenting are older and often much more ill. Therefore in general the outcomes measures of such therapy have been shown to be inferior to that of men in many studies. But final outcomes seem to be comparable in women and men. In the past balloon angioplasty and stenting was considered more risky in women. But the latest evidence corrects this misnomer by demonstrating that women in-fact do very well after this form of treatment.

More men get bay pass surgery than women. It has been observed that women fair less well after bypass surgery. Many different causes seem to contribute to this situation.

Very remarkable differences have been observed in the rates of participation of women in cardiac rehabilitation after a heart attack or after coronary artery bypass surgery. Cardiac rehabilitation has been demonstrated to be very useful in reducing mortality rates and preventing recurrent heart attacks. As was the case with Simone less women participate in cardiac rehabilitation therefore less women benefit from this lifesaving form of treatment. The reasons for this situation are many. Doctors and other health care workers seem to refer less women for cardiac rehabilitation. Even those who get referred fail to commence on the program and those who somehow get started seem to drop out early. Household chores and paucity of transportation or lack of access have been identified as major impediments to women's participation in rehabilitation programs. Women of minority groups and low socio-economic status seem to be the most affected by these limitations.

Women and coronary risk factors

Risk factor modification to prevent heart disease among women still is not widely practiced. Once again the main reason for this is the traditional notion that heart disease was a disease affecting men only. Researchers have identified some major ways the risk factors for heart disease differ between men and women.

The commonest coronary risk factor among women is physical inactivity. Diabetes is more important as a coronary risk factor among women than men. Obesity too is relatively more prevalent among women than men. Relative importance of high blood pressure and high cholesterol levels in women has been observed to be less than in men. However, trials on secondary prevention of heart attacks have demonstrated that strict control of high blood pressure and blood cholesterol levels can prevent heart attacks in women, particularly in those who also have diabetes. Smoking is fast becoming a major risk factor among women as more men seem to give up smoking while more women seem to take it up. Increasing numbers of young women take up smoking cigarettes and this trend has caused serious concerns among doctors. This is of particular significance in that unlike men, women find it harder to quit the habit and get over the addiction. This is so even with treatment. Women need maximum possible treatment when attempting to quit. Combination of behavioral treatment, and the drug Zyban (burpropion) together with the nicotine patch seem to produce the best results.

Women who suffer from polycystic ovary syndrome as discussed above are at very high risk of heart disease. These women in addition to developing multiple cysts in the ovaries have the combination of cardiac risk factors of abdominal obesity, high blood pressure, diabetes and high cholesterol levels. They have a resistance in their body to the activity of the hormone insulin that regulates blood sugar levels. The combination of above abnormalities, also called the “insulin resistance metabolic syndrome” places the woman with this condition at high risk of heart disease.

On a positive note in general women seem to have higher levels of the good cholesterol HDL than men. Many trials looking into the effects of physical exercise have confirmed the benefits of regular physical activity in the prevention of the first heart attack and recurrent heart attacks in women.

Do women have different symptoms?

Very often women do not present with typical symptoms of chest pain when having a heart attack. But however, the vast majority of women suffering a heart attack in fact present with typical chest pain. The prodromal or the fore warning symptoms that women experience can often be different to that of men. Most women experience excessive fatigue or discomfort of the upper abdomen that could easily be mistaken for gastritis or reflux pain as was the case with Simone. Some others may experience persistent nausea and vomiting. It has been noticed that very often women suppress their symptoms and thus present late. In addition when women present with heart attacks they are more often misdiagnosed. This may explain why more women compared to men die of their first heart attack.

However the converse is true too. Compared to men the chest pain women experience is more often not due to heart disease. Therefore in younger women even a positive stress test cannot accurately predict the existence of heart disease. However when women develop heart disease their outcome is always worse than that of men. Mortality and long term disability due to heart disease is much higher among women.

Hormone replacement therapy

For a while doctors were led to believe that hormone replacement therapy was a miracle agent that protected women from developing heart disease. Hormone replacement therapy for women after menopause helps with the symptoms of menopause such as hot flashes. It also has proven value in the prevention and treatment of osteoporosis. Going by the evidence from observational studies doctors believed that hormone replacement afforded a very powerful protective effects from heart disease. For a considerable time doctors actively prescribed combined estrogen and progestin tablets to women with the aim of preventing heart disease. But these studies were flawed as realized later, due to a factor called the "healthy user bias". Healthy user bias occurs due to healthier and health conscious women taking hormone replacement therapy compared sicker women that did not. So the group that took hormone replacement therapy was much healthier to start with. Thus their long-term outlook appeared better than those who did not take the treatment. This difference was falsely attributed to the treatment with hormone replacement while the real reason remained the disparity of health in the two groups prior to taking the therapy.

Recently two well designed randomized controlled trial shed real light into this misconception. In these two trials called the Women's Health Initiative and HERS (Heart and Estrogen/Progestin Replacement Study) researchers demonstrated that hormone replacement therapy did not offer any protection from heart disease. The former study proved that hormone therapy was of no use in the prevention of the first heart attack (primary prevention) and the second study proved that it was also useless in the prevention of recurrent heart attacks (secondary prevention). In fact they observed more harmful effects in the way of increased heart attacks in some instances and also increased incidence of clots in the veins (venous thrombosis) and strokes among those who took hormone treatment.

Hormone replacement in the long term was contributing to the development of cancers of the breast and the uterus. Therefore the current recommendation is hormone replacement therapy only for relief from menopausal symptoms. It is recommended that it should not be continued beyond the first year after menopause.

What women should do

Women in general are less physically active. Rates of involvement in physical exercise are very low among women and this is a major contributing factor to the high prevalence of life style oriented disorders among women. It is important that physical exercise be promoted among women on a wider scale. Creation of non-threatening environments such as women only gyms and exercise groups has been suggested as practical solutions to this problem by some experts. Doctors too should take a greater interest and initiative in promoting and facilitating physical activity among the female clientele.

Evidence to the beneficial effects of physical exercise to women is overwhelming. A large study recently revealed that half hour of walking at least three times a week could reduce the risk of women of all ages getting heart attacks by 50%.

Measures at obesity reduction among women too are of great importance. Obesity seems to be reaching epidemic proportions among the poor and the minority women. It has been observed that the effect of exercise on weight reduction and maintenance is not as efficient among women as it is among men. Therefore exercise together with diet and other means should be combined in achieving weight loss goals among women.

Diabetes is more important as a cardiac risk factor among women. Diabetes is of further significance in that it negates the relative protection that pre-menopausal women have against heart disease. Thus diabetic women suffer heart attacks at a younger age. Obesity and physical inactivity are major contributors to the development of diabetes among women. Once again diabetes is more prevalent among the poor and the minority women.

Just as in men good control of high blood pressure reduces heart attacks in women. The exact relationship between cholesterol lowering and prevention of heart disease is not as clear in women as it is in men. This is due to the fact that the majority of the trials investigating the benefits of cholesterol lowering therapy did not include adequate numbers of women. However there is evidence to suggest the benefits of cholesterol lowering among women.

Smoking is emerging as a major coronary risk factor among women. Majority of the heart attacks in younger women occur among smokers. Women find it difficult to give up smoking due to the stronger psychological dependence associated with the habit.

It is hoped that the concerted efforts currently underway to increase awareness of heart disease among women would help control this growing health concern.

Chapter 10

Making love to the heart's content -Sex and the heart

Ben is a character and every time he comes to see me in my clinic I get to have an enjoyable conversation. He was 60 and an ex-US Marine corps sergeant. He often shares with me his philosophical overviews of different contemporary issues ranging from politics to entertainment. He has also told me various fact filled stories of his adventure filled days in the military while stationed overseas. One memorable highlight was his visit to Sydney harbor aboard an aircraft carrier in the 1960s. "All we did there was eating, drinking and having sex" he chuckled with a twinkle in his eye. But recently during a regular consultation I realized that Ben was not his usual self. He was seemingly troubled by some thing.

Ben has had coronary heart disease for a few years. I have treated him previously with cardiac catheterization with good results. He also has blockages in other arteries outside of his heart. Two years ago he developed a nagging pain in his legs, particularly in the calf area upon walking. This pain would disappear upon resting for a few minutes. When I examined him on that occasion I realized that the pulse in his feet could barely be felt. What Ben had at that time was "*intermittent claudication*" in other words inadequate blood supply to his legs due to obstructions in the arteries that carry blood to the legs. This is like angina of the leg muscles – developing pain due to inadequate blood supply. Once I confirmed my diagnosis by angiograms of his legs I treated him by unblocking the arteries through catheterization. Ben has done well since and he has been claudication free ever since. But the fact remained that he had problems of blood vessels in many parts of his body. In medical terms he was a "*vasculopath*" or a person with blocks in many arteries of the body. He had blocks in the arteries that supply blood to his genitalia too. Due to this he was impotent. Ben wanted to be sexually active. I prescribed him *Viagra* upon making sure that it was safe for him to take and that he was not on any other drugs that can have harmful interactions. His impotence was very well managed with *Viagra*.

However Ben has started to experience some chest pain on walking a few blocks since about three months ago. His internist has started him on a nitrate tablet that helped to alleviate this angina. Going on the nitrate meant that he could not take *Viagra* any more! *Viagra* and nitrate are a deadly combination. Having no sex since starting the nitrate was what made Ben so depressed and frustrated. I had to get him off the nitrate and the way to do this was to treat the blocked coronary that could be causing his angina.

I performed a coronary angiogram on Ben few days later. He had a critical narrowing in the right coronary and that was causing the angina. I went on to treat him by placing a drug coated stent across the blocked segment of the artery. Ben's angina was fixed! And he no longer required the nitrate. I did an exercise stress test to ensure that he did not develop angina on exertion anymore. Then I could safely stop the nitrate completely and start him back on his much-anticipated *Viagra* tablet. I could see the happiness written all over Ben's face when I handed him the prescription for the tablet. Ben had his usual twinkle back in his eye!

Heart and Sex

There have been many observations made on the relationship between sexual activity and heart disease. Sexual activity is a form of physical exertion that can place a considerable demand on your heart. Many questions arise about the association between sex and heart. What is the significance of the physical demand associated with sex? Can sex overwhelm your heart so as to trigger a heart attack? How much of a strain does sexual activity put your heart at? Is the level of physical exertion associated with sexual activity too much for the heart of a patient at risk of sustaining a heart attack?

Doctors tried to answer these questions by measuring the strain on the heart during sexual activity of a group of volunteers. These volunteers involved in sexual activity while being monitored for heart activity. The scientists found out that during sex heart rate and blood pressure certainly increased in a similar manner to that during physical activity. But this degree of increase in heart's activity was not too severe. So they concluded that demand on the heart during sex to be of moderated degree. Their observations showed that highest demand and strain on the heart was during orgasmic phase of the sexual act. They described the total physical demand on the heart during sex to be similar in magnitude to that during a game of tennis.

What the scientists researching into the effects of sex on the heart have uncovered is interesting as well as reassuring. Their work has demonstrated that sexual activity involves only a moderate degree of physical exertion. This too only for a relatively short duration. So they concluded that sex does not put too much of a burden on ones heart and the risk of having a heart attack during sex is not too high. But it should be stressed that their still is some risk. Your risk of a heart attack during sex should be estimated by discussing the topic with your doctor.

Heart attack during sex

What is the risk of your having a heart attack during sexual activity? To shed light to this question, scientists studied a series of patients admitted to hospital with heart attack. They inquired each patient to ascertain what they had been doing in the immediate time period before the onset of the heart attack. In this study scientists discovered that only about 1% of the patients have had sex prior to the onset of their heart attack. It was also revealed that the first two hours after sexual activity is the period of increased risk for heart attacks.

Improving your physical fitness can help decrease your risk of having a heart attack during sex. Moderate degree of physical exercise regularly has been demonstrated to be useful in decreasing this risk. Scientists demonstrated that those who exercise regularly had lesser increases in the heart rate and the blood pressure during sex. This means these individuals placed less of a strain on their hearts during sex.

Doctors can identify those at risk of heart attacks during sex by performing an exercise stress test. They have found out that changes in heart activity and changes suggesting the possible risk of heart attack during an exercise stress test accurately predicted what would happen to the heart during sex. Thus doctors can identify those at risk and manage them accordingly to prevent the possible heart attack that could be triggered by sex.

Sudden death during sex

What is the risk of sudden death due to a heart attack or cardiac arrest during sex? There have been case reports of extremely rare incidents of players dropping dead while taking part in sports. Since sex is a form of physical activity that places a strain on the heart it is important to look at any potential risks of sudden death during sex. Not many studied have been carried out in this specific area of significant interest. There is only a single study that is quoted often in the medical literature that deals with this topic. This study was carried out in Japan in the sixties. In this study the scientists showed that only 0.6% of the sudden deaths in the studied series of sudden deaths happened during sex. Out of these deaths the vast majority had happened while married men were having sex with partners other than their wives. So it was concluded that the risk of sudden death during sex is extremely low. Anxiety provoking situations surrounding the sexual activity such as extramarital sex may increase this risk but only by a small degree. But the findings of this study have been subject to much criticism due to some fundamental scientific and statistical flaws that some say, are associated with the study.

Sex in fact is good for the heart

Is regular sexual activity beneficial to your heart just like regular physical activity? To answer this question scientists studied a group of middle-aged individuals over a period of ten years. At the end of the ten years they found out that those who had sex more often lived longer than those who had less sex. They also showed that a higher frequency of orgasms decreased ones chance of dying from heart disease or to that matter, of any cause. In fact high frequency of sex and orgasms decreased the chance of dying from any cause by almost 50%. So it seems that sex is good for the heart. And more sex may prolong your life expectancy.

Sexual dysfunction and heart disease

Erectile dysfunction or impotence is frequently associated with coronary heart disease. Those with heart disease have a high prevalence of impotence and those with impotence have a high incidence of heart disease. The very mechanism that gives rise to blocks in the coronary arteries is known to cause blocks in the arteries supplying the penis too thus the two diseases have a common kinship. Both are disorders of the inner lining or the endothelium of the arteries.

In addition some of the drugs that are used to treat heart disease and blood pressure can cause erectile dysfunction as a side effect. Heart failure and heart attacks can give rise to impotence. The impotence associated with these conditions could be due to the physical effects of the disease as well as the associated anxiety and depression too. Is there a risk to the heart associated with the resumption of sexual activity in those who have been successfully treated for erectile dysfunction? The risk of sexual activity associated cardiovascular risk is considered very small even in those who resume sexual activity after a period of abstinence due to impotence.

Doctors are encouraged to probe into the existence of impotence in patients being treated for heart disease. It is known that despite successful treatment of heart disease the patient may continue to have a compromised quality of life due to non-addressed impotence.

PDE5I treatment for impotence

Impotence can happen due to many causes. The most common causes include diabetes, psychological reasons, disease of small blood vessels, nerve disease, disease of the penis it self and prostate surgery. Impotence due to all these causes can be very effectively treated with a class of drugs that is scientifically known as phospodiesterase 5 inhibitors or PDE5Is.

There are three forms of this drug available in the market world over (some countries may not have all three approved for sale as yet). They are sildenafil (Viagra), tadalafil (Cialis), and vardenafil (Levitra). They have demonstrated good efficacy, good tolerance by consumers and safety in several well-controlled clinical trials. There is no evidence to suggest any increased risk of heart attack brought about by PDE5Is. These drugs may start acting as early as within 15 minutes after taking. The majority that takes the drug achieved an erection within 30 minutes of taking the tablet. The effect of the drug can last anywhere up to 24 hours and beyond. PDE5Is have been in use for more than five years and there is lots of information to its efficacy, side effects as well risks associated with its use. Major side effects, though not very common include headache, flushing and indigestion. Only less than 2% of the users had to discontinue the use of the drug and this was mainly due to headaches. In general these drugs have proven to be very effective, safe and well tolerated if taken according to prescription guidelines and doctors advice.

Both younger and older individuals showed similar response to the drug. It was very effective in helping to secure erection and also thus significantly improve the quality of life of those taking the drug.

Dangers of PDE5Is

This drug acts by expanding the arteries of the body. As a result of this action your blood pressure can drop. This potential for dropping the blood pressure is the major risk associated with this drug. What is the real risk?

There have been case reports of fatal drug interaction when PDE5Is were taken together with nitrate drugs given for angina. This combination leads to a profound drop in blood pressure that can kill the person. So it is strictly advised that PDE5Is and nitrates should not be taken together. Another class of high blood pressure medications called alpha blockers too can interact with PDE5Is when taken at the same time, leading to significant drops in the blood pressure. Therefore these agents too should not be taken together. All patients on medications for angina and high blood pressure should review their medications with the doctors prior to commencing PDE5I therapy for impotence. Doctor's advice on prescription should be strictly adhered to.

Diabetes and PDE5I therapy

Diabetes is one of the major causes of sexual dysfunction and impotence in our community. PDE5Is have been observed to be effective in most diabetics no matter what other diabetes related complication they had. The levels of control of blood sugar levels or the type of diabetes one has had no impact on the efficacy of the drug in controlling and treating impotence.

Female sexuality and PDE5I treatment

Sexual dysfunction is very common among females and this incidence seems to increase with advancing age. The role and efficacy of PDE5I agents in treating female sexual dysfunction has been an area of interest among medical researchers. But no conclusive results have become available as yet to suggest any benefits of this agent to the female patient. PDE5I is known to act in female clitoral tissue and the potential for its use to stimulate female sexual arousal remains a potential possibility. It may have a role to play in increasing clitoral sensitivity and vaginal lubrication and enhancing of arousal by these means.

Chapter 11

Treasures of the East – Yoga for good health

One hot summer night, during my medical residency a few years ago, I had one of the strangest encounters ever in my whole life. It was indeed a close brush with the paranormal. I was stationed at the hospital in beautiful Byron Bay about 600 miles north of Sydney along the eastern coastal belt of Australia. If I do not share with you a little bit of what is so special about Byron bay first, my story would not be complete. Byron bay is world renown for its spectacular natural beauty. Its endless stretches of sun kissed golden beaches are havens for sun seekers and the gracious waves off the coast heaven sent to the avid surfers. In addition the beach-front is interrupted by gigantic rock formations that at some places extend into the sea as rocky points. From atop these rocky peaks one can glimpse in the far away ocean, migrating sperm whales and native schools of dolphins frolicking in sheer glee. The weather here is rather warm round the year. Little in-lands there are the thick rain forests of Mullambimby where wild parties take place every full moon night. The rolling green hills of Bungalow few miles in-lands from the bay are breathtakingly beautiful and a drive-through is immensely relaxing to any stressed out and weary mind.

Byron bay was obscure farmland when it was discovered by the hippies in the late sixties and the early seventies. First the area became an epicenter for the flower generation and many communities for the love makers sprang up in the vicinity. Vegetarian colonies and agri-farm communities of the Hare-Krishna movement also set up camp there. In the eighties Byron bay transformed rapidly from the hippie haven to a popular tourist destination with its beach front properties becoming prime possessions of the rich and the famous as well as the international hoteliers.

Byron bay how ever still remains an attraction to the followers of the new age movement. There exist organic-vegan communities, health resorts and of course nude colonies. Often one can encounter a seeker of enlightenment meditating in some tranquil beach front far-removed from the popular tourist areas, coming face to face with nature that is unadulterated and untouched. Some say that Byron bay is one of the focal centers of earth where cosmic energy flows uninterrupted and concentrated and that one can tune into the vibes of the vast universe here. Machu-pichu in Peru, the Himalayan mountains and the beaches of Bali are considered by them as some of the other such places of energy flow elsewhere in the world.

I was rostered to be one of the two emergency room doctors that night. It was a quiet and long night where not much activity took place as usual. My colleague opted to take a short snooze in the on-call room while I held the fort armed with my mug of freshly brewed coffee. Suddenly the "bat-phone", the dedicated phone for the emergency medical teams and ambulance crew started to ring breaking the eerie silence. As I picked up the receiver I could hear the anxious voice of the paramedic from the other end. He was describing to me a middle-aged man picked up from a beach-front cottage. He had been unconscious and non-breathing with a weak and very slow pulse when the paramedics arrived at the scene. They quickly inserted a tube into his windpipe and started artificial ventilation. Despite multiple injections of atropine and adrenaline, his heart rate had not picked up and the paramedic had commenced chest compressions as they could not record a satisfactory blood pressure. There was no evidence of trauma, excess alcohol intake or illicit drug use. The patient had no history of epileptic fits and his blood sugar levels were normal – thus ruling out the possible common causes of such presentations. They reported of a Glasgow coma scale score for the patient of 7 to 8 – suggesting near death or virtual death!

The next moment I was getting prepared to receive the patient since the ambulance was still a good twenty minutes away from the hospital. My expectations were not high and, in the back of my mind, I was ready to certify death on arrival as it was very likely to be the case with what I have heard so far from the ambulance. I called the on-call anesthesiologist and the cardiologist. I donned my gloves, scrubs and face-mask while my assisting nurses prepared the equipment and the resuscitation bay bed for the impending arrival. It felt like a long wait and the on-call physicians soon arrived and got ready for the resuscitation process.

The ambulance soon rolled in and its two back doors swung open. And the automatic glass door of the ambulance bay opened simultaneously. My heart was thumping with the adrenaline rush and I could see the solemn and resolved faces of my other colleagues all well prepared to jump into action. I could not believe my eyes with what I saw next.

The "near-dead" patient suddenly sat up, pulled the ventilating tube off his mouth and started smiling with an expression of amazement written all over his face. Spell bound were my self, all my crew and of course the ambulance crew that were frenetically trying to resuscitate the man all this while. We all were speechless for a moment. "What is happening, where am I?" the patient broke the silence. We all were dumb founded. This was miraculous. I have never seen or heard of anyone springing back to almost normal self with no treatment after being ventilated and kept on basic life support. Usually patients that arrive in such a state would be very ill. If resuscitated successfully, they would be transferred to the intensive care unit for further supportive therapy. Even if a remediable cause for the illness was found, the patient is expected only to make a rather slow and prolonged recovery in the intensive care unit with full life support.

We soon establish that the patient was clinically stable with good blood pressure and good oxygenation of his blood. The next few minutes were spent explaining to him what has taken place since the time he became unconscious. Then I went on to obtain a formal medical history from him and perform a detailed physical examination. Upon the conclusion of my clinical assessment of him I could not find anything wrong at all.

Let me call him Max. Max was 51 years old. He denied any

symptom or discomfort at that time in fact he was feeling very well. He denied having any past medical condition of any significance and also denied alcohol consumption or illicit drug use. He was a very friendly man with good common sense. He was an investment banker from London and was holidaying in Byron bay with his partner Betty. He has been yoga practitioner for over twenty years and has been visiting places round the world where according to him "concentrations of cosmic energy flows are found" to practice yoga and to meditate. Early that night he has been practicing "Tantric yoga" and meditating with his partner. He made the most bizarre and amazing claim at this point. He had been awakening his "charkas" through meditation and yoga. Betty, who also was an experienced yoga practitioner, has been assisting him. While she was stimulating his "*muladhara charka*" located at the tip of the spine, where according to him the boundless form of personal energy called "*kundalini energy*" lies, he had experienced an amazing awakening and a feeling of absolute bliss. He has felt detachment from his body and attained a state of levitation. He was in this state till he woke up in the emergency room. He was totally oblivious to all what has happened in between.

At this point Betty chipped in with what she observed. Betty was about 39 years old and has been practicing yoga and meditation for almost ten years. She has been stimulating the focal point situated at the root of Max's spinal column with gentle pressure while Max was in deep meditation in a yoga posture. After some time into the exercise Betty noticed that Max had stopped breathing. She quickly stopped her activity and checked his pulse and could not detect any. Then she started calling Max by his name and shaking him in case he was in deep sleep. Having had no response she had thumped on his chest several times as per the basic resuscitation protocol. With no effect she had commenced mouth-to-mouth breathing and chest compressions. In between she has taken a brief moment to call the emergency 911 for help. Emergency medial team arrived few minutes later and took over the resuscitation process.

The story was unbelievable and intriguing. It certainly defied any scientific or medical explanation. Max and Betty requested discharge from the hospital. But I opted to keep him in the ER under observation for at least six more hours. Meanwhile all his blood test results came back as being normal. The blood and urine drug screen was negative. After close monitoring for six hours I discharged Max from the hospital the next morning. However the impact of this incident remained with me for a long time to come. The discussions I had with my senior, more experienced medical colleagues or the research I did into the relevant medical literature shed disappointingly little light into the phenomenon I witnessed. At this point I decided to seek more information about the ancient practices of the east and physical and medical effects of theirs by consulting experienced practitioners and reading authoritative literature. This also involved traveling to Asia and the Indian sub continent. It is a journey of discovery that has been very revealing and still continuing.

The traditional practices of the east such as yoga, meditation, ayurveda, tai chi etc. seem to hold some keys to healthy living and the control of body processes both physiological and biochemical. Though not scientifically studied in depth, increasingly more light is shed into the physiological effects and the health benefits of such practices. Yoga, meditation and tai- chi are increasingly put into scientific testing and interesting information has been uncovered. Some such revelations have been published in reputed medical journals. In the following chapters I have endeavored to review some scientific information into the benefits of some traditional eastern practices in the realms of cardiac health and prevention of heart disease. While these research did not help me uncover the enigma surrounding my Byron bay experience it certainly exposed me to the treasure trove of Eastern practices beneficial for heart health and the treatment of heart disease.

Tantric yoga is one branch of the vast eastern scientific tradition called "Yoga Shastra" or the discipline of yoga. Yoga is very popular. Many things have been said and written about yoga. There are many claims to its efficacy in bringing about stress relief and relaxation. In addition there is the occasional report on the general health benefits of yoga. Expert yoga teachers both eastern and western have exciting and interesting facts to share about yoga. Such claims are often substantiated by complementary healers and allied health practitioners. But what does your doctor say about yoga? You may say…"not much" or "nothing at all!". The fact is many doctors do not know much about the holistic or mind-body methods of medical therapy such as yoga, meditation, ayurveda etc. But the truth is yoga is in reality an effective health practice as claimed by those who teach and advocate it. Scientific research too seems to back these claims. To make your journey of discovery into good and healthy living complete and perfectly balanced, you too should know the scientific truths about the holistic practices such as yoga. Such essential knowledge may help integrate these practices into your lifestyle and reap their benefits to help you live a healthier and fuller life.

Modern discovery of an ancient tradition

Yoga is an ancient and rich tradition of physical and mental exercise that is used to generate and propagate mental and physical well-being. It is also a therapeutic practice that brings about healing through the harmonization of the mental, physical and spiritual faculties of the human being. Its origins date back to prehistoric times. Though physical and mental practices similar to yoga have been identified with many ancient cultures and nations, it is in India that Yoga prevailed and flourished as a living tradition. The popular types of yoga mainly present as forms of physical exercise or meditation. However the essential and real yoga is a complex philosophy with many diverse concepts and practices. Over thousands of years traditional medical practitioners of India and

Asia used various elements of yoga to treat and prevent illness and uphold good health. Many traditional chronicles and historical accounts testify to the incredible good health and longevity enjoyed by dedicated yoga practitioners.

As yoga began to get popular in the west there were many anecdotal accounts that emerged to claim its health benefits. The benefits of conventional exercise to cardiovascular health and well-being have been scientifically proven. The life saving cardiovascular benefits of regular physical exercise was further proven by observational and clinical trials. In a similar manner scientists and researchers have also tested yoga. One early such study was published in the prestigious medical journal, Lancet, where the ability of a yoga practitioner to control heart rate voluntarily was discussed. There were also reports about the ability of expert yoga practitioners from the Himalayas to control their body temperature and emit heat to the out side environment. In one such experiment scientists observed scantily clad yoga practitioners meditating in freezing temperatures while snow melted around them due to the heat emitted. As the physiological responses such as heart rate, blood pressure, body temperature are regulated by the body's autonomic nervous system we usually have no control over them. Scientists who studied the yoga practitioners were amazed to discover how through meditation and the practice of yoga these individuals could bring autonomic neurological functions under their voluntary control. Scientists from the very early days of research into yoga speculated a mechanism of mind body integration associated with its practice whereby one could control autonomous body functions to prevent and treat diseases.

With the scientific validation of the health benefits of yoga, its value and relevance as a means of alternative or complementary therapy is becoming gradually recognized. However it has a very wide acceptance as a popular and established means of recreation and relaxation. I believe that yoga may have a far greater role to play in the contemporary health care scene. When established protocols in medicine are increasingly advocating the use of multiple forms of drugs and expensive interventions as the standard of therapy, one has to be mindful of the associated adverse effects, dangers as well as their sky rocketing costs. This is particularly so in the prevention and the treatment of heart disease. I strongly believe with reason that integration of practices such as yoga may well compliment the protocols of modern cardiovascular medicine in such a way that the combination would yield better health outcomes and drastically cut the costs.

What is Yoga?

Adoption of a range of very simple to quite complex postures called "*asanas*" (the Sanskrit word for seat) and maintaining such adopted postures for specified durations are the corner stones of yoga practice. But this is only a part of the process. The next most important aspect of yoga is the controlled breathing technique called "*pranayama*" breathing. (meaning "life-breath" in Sanskrit). The third component of the yoga practice is meditation or "*dhyana*". The yogic meditation is a very wide and complex topic. However there are some basic techniques of meditation that are simple and practical and that can be practiced without any in-depth involvement. One such meditational form involves the recital of a simple syllable. The most commonly used syllable is "*om*" (pronounced as aum) which is the sound of the universe or the cosmic resonance according to ancient Indian philosophy. Repeated recitation of this word is said to harmonize your mind and body with the energy waves of the abysmal universe where matter and energy exist in unification. Fourth and the most complex component of yoga involve the "cleansing practices" or "*kriyas*". These cleansing practices are meant to clean your nose and the air passages, stomach and the gastrointestinal tract.

The practical forms of everyday yoga are quite simple to follow and even to master. The simplicity as well as the remarkable mental and physical benefits it brings has made this ancient tradition extremely popular in our modern society. Its popularity is so high that yoga has become a fad or a fashion item.

History of yoga

Experts have identified yoga to be more than five thousand years old. It is believed to have originated in the earliest of human civilizations that arose in the banks of the mighty Indus river in southern-central Asia. At first yoga was handed over from generation to generation as a living tradition and a spiritual practice. The first written records of yoga are found in the ancient textbook called "*Yoga Sutra*". This is believed to have been written around 200 BC and 300 AD. It was written by the earliest known authority on yoga, a Hindu philosopher or a guru called Patanjali. Since then over the years many such teachers have developed and changed the various traditions of yoga. Some remained to be handed over the generations by popular lore and others by means of texts. A Hindu missionary by the name of Swami Vivekananda introduced yoga to the west in the late nineteenth century. Till then yoga remained an exclusive domain of the priestly Brahmin cast of India.

The body postures (Asanas)

The fundamental element of yoga involves adoption of postures or *asanas* and maintaining such postures while practicing controlled breathing and mental concentration. According to the ancient classic on yoga called the *Gherananda Samhita* there are over 840000 different postures in yoga. But it goes on to recommend 32 postures as being suitable for regular practice by the general public. Each posture symbolizes a phenomenon from nature. This symbolism highlights the balance of elements that is the very essence of yoga practice. Just as everything in nature exists and persists in a perpetual state of perfect balance, the yoga postures are meant to mirror and adopt such natural balance. The main objective of adopting yoga postures is the restoration of that natural balance within you. The same text advices to maintain each posture for periods of 5-20 yogic breaths at a time.

Yoga breathing is called *pranayama* breathing. It involves slow-

deep inspiration through the nose with the use of diaphragmatic and abdominal muscles. At full inspiration the breath is held momentarily. Then it is exhaled very slowly. Once again the respiration is paused momentarily at full expiration. You are to be completely mindful of your breathing. As you inhale you should mentally picture air entering your body though your nostrils and as you breath deeper, visualize in your mind your body filling with life giving, energizing (air contains oxygen that help burn body fuels to generate energy) and purifying (air help remove many waste material from your body in the blood-lung interphase) air. And then you exhale in a similar manner with complete mindfulness. Your mind thus should be focused completely on your inhaling and exhaling of each breath. Thus your mind is cleared, purified and rested in a rhythmic stillness. This form of yogic meditational breathing is called the "*anapana sathi*" or "*uggayi*". The mental relaxation such breathing techniques bring about can sooth any degree of mental and physical stress. What is more exciting about this is that it can be done any time anywhere under any circumstance - without necessarily having to adopt a specific yoga posture. For example I know of people who overcame road rage and stress of driving in busy streets of the city by practicing *pranayama* breathing while driving!
The relaxation that results from this type of soothing breathing will bring down your heart rate and blood pressure thus helping to prevent heart disease and the triggering of heart attacks.

Restoration to the cosmic rhythm

A recent article in a well-known medical journal described how mindfulness based stress reduction decreased the average number of visits to the doctor's office in the inner city areas of the US. Stressors of urban life have been identified as being directly causative of many physical and mental illnesses including coronary heart disease. Mind-body stress management techniques such as yoga can contribute to good health and prevention of heart attacks according observational scientific studies.

The whole nature from the fathomless universe to the subatomic particle is in a fine equilibrium. This equilibrium is the result of a natural rhythm. In nature, everything happens according to this finely balanced rhythm. According to the ancient philosophy, this balance of rhythm is the key to wholeness. Restoration of this natural balance and the rhythm thereof is the way to healthy living. According to the most advanced research carried out into the physiology and pathology of heart disease and risk factors for heart disease it is the disruption of the natural rhythmic variability in your heart rate and blood pressure that contributes to the development of heart disease. In medicine it is called the natural heart rate variability and baro-reflex sensitivity. Researchers have demonstrated that these natural rhythms of the body disrupted by our busy and unhealthy life styles can be restored by practicing the slow breathing techniques of yoga. Recently European researchers compared the physiological effects of the recital of yoga mantra "*om*" and the recital of the catholic holy rosary. They demonstrated that by both means your respiration could be slowed down to 6 breaths per minute. Practising this slow and rhythmic breathing could to restore heart rate variability and baro reflex sensitivity in the people who were tested. The beneficial effects of this kind of rhythmic breathing was seen with the improvements in the electrical activity of the heart, in the blood pressure as well as in the blood flow signals to the brain.

Can Yoga Prevent Heart Attacks?

Some remarkable medical and scientific research carried out in the US, Europe and India has shed light to this question. According to the results of these investigations the practice of yoga is very effective in controlling many of your coronary risk factors. Some times it was seen that even a short course of yoga exercises could have powerful effects that were as potent as drug therapy. With the safe and effective control of coronary risk factors doctors showed that heart disease could be prevented. Thus regular practice of yoga has scientifically confirmed benefits in the prevention of heart disease. In controlled trials doctors demonstrated that those that practiced yoga suffered heart attacks more rarely.

High blood pressure

High blood pressure is one of the most common coronary risk factors. It is also a risk factor for non -coronary heart failure, stroke and kidney failure. The best and the most potent way to control blood pressure is through drug therapy. Simple life style changes alone can bring blood pressure down, but only by a lesser degree. For example a 100mmol/day reduction in sodium intake can lower your blood pressure by 5 mmHg systolic and 3mmHg diastolic. A similar magnitude reduction in the blood pressure is effected by performing conventional aerobic exercise for 30-45 minutes a day on 4-5 days a week at a moderate intensity (50% of maximum effort or oxygen consumption- as in brisk walking). A research project that compared drug therapy, yoga and life style changes such as reducing salt consumption etc. in a head to head manner showed that practicing yoga one hour a day for eleven weeks was as effective as taking drugs to control your blood pressure. And it was far more effective than life style changes alone. Therefore one can comfortably conclude that simple life style measures combined with the regular practice of yoga can control your blood pressure more effectively than even drug therapy. Taking into consideration the staggering costs and the side effects of drugs, the combined life style adjustment and yoga approach seem more desirable.
Many other clinical trials and physiological studies have shown that conventional exercise in combination with programmed relaxation by means of biofeedback, psychotherapy or transcendental meditation can have profound blood pressure controlling effect.

How does yoga control your blood pressure? Scientists have shown that yoga can restore your body's natural rhythms and equilibrium. Due to the effects of modern life style your natural balances are disrupted to such an extent that your body's sensitivity to the natural rhythms is lost. The main cause behind high blood pressure is your body's insensitivity to the signals generated by the constant changes in your blood pressure. This is called 'baroreflex insensitivity" as we have discussed before. The root cause for this situation is the malfunctioning of your autonomic nervous system. If your autonomic nerve function is intact your body can detect the fluctuations of your blood pressure and make necessary changes to your heart's contractions and the tone of the muscles lining your arteries to regulate the pressure. In other words, you have natural protection from high blood pressure if your autonomic nervous system is working well. Yoga seems to be effective in restoring your autonomic nervous function and thus re-establishing the baroreflex sensitivity. Restoration of your body's natural balance has the ability to restore the disruptions caused by this imbalance.

Thus we can appreciate that yoga acts by restoring a natural and normal regulatory function in your body. Therefore yoga can be identified as a natural remedy for high blood pressure. The yoga postures that involve the adoption of a head down-body up tilt such as "*sarvangasana*" has been identified to be particularly effective in the control of blood pressure. Researchers noted that even after a short 3-week course of yoga they could identify favourable changes in the brain waves (improvements in the alpha index of the EEG) and neurochemical levels in the blood. These changes were very suggestive of improved autonomic neurological function.

Medical scientists discovered that yoga not only could control high blood pressure but also reverse the cardiac complications that result from long standing high blood pressure. Long standing blood pressure can cause enlargement of the heart walls and this can lead to cardiac failure. Even after a short duration such as two week's practice of yoga could reverse the enlargement of the heart that was due to long standing high blood pressure. This change in the heart wall thickness of the participants of the study was confirmed by repeated echocardiograms.

Yoga's effect on cholesterol level and body weight

Excess body weight and obesity is associated with many illnesses that include heart disease and high blood pressure. It increases your mortality significantly. Losing weight is often very challenging and at times even very expensive. Many find it difficult to get involved in physical exercise that helps burn calories and thus cause weight loss. Interestingly a group of researchers that studied various treatment strategies for obesity discovered that regular practice of yoga had profound weight loss effects. They divided a group of obese individuals to two sub groups. One group practiced yoga regularly for a year while the other group did not. All other factors including the diet were kept essentially similar in the two groups. After a year the yoga group had lost weight significantly while the control group had not. Yet another group of researchers in a separate experiment showed significant weight loss in individuals who practiced yoga and meditation for three months in a residential setting.

Another beneficial effect of yoga is its ability to reduce cholesterol level in your blood. Wight loss and cholesterol lowering effects of yoga cannot be due to excess calorie burning alone because the simple practice of yoga asanas does not involve the rapid repetitive movement of large muscles that use large amounts of energy.

Yoga for diabetes

Researchers also studied the effects of yoga on diabetes. A group of diabetic patients on medications to control blood sugar levels, who practiced yoga under experimental conditions showed significant improvements in their level of blood sugar control. As the program progressed they required less medication to control blood sugar levels. Yoga has been shown to be a simple and economical treatment method that may be considered to be a beneficial addition for diabetic patients. The exact mechanism by which yoga acts to control blood sugar level is still not conclusively identified.

What does yoga do to your body?

Excessive unbalanced activity of the neurological system and the hormonal system of your body (neurohormonal system) has been identified as a main factor that increases your risk of developing coronary heart disease. This may explain how the lifestyle factors come together to become a major risk factor for heart disease. The level of activity of your neurohormonal system can be measured by checking various neurochemical and hormone levels in your blood and the levels of their breakdown products in your urine. Researchers studied these blood and urine markers of neurohormonal activity in subjects who practiced yoga for a set period of time. They reported that their neurohormonal activity was decreased upon completing the yoga program. Their urinary excretion of substances such as epinephrine, norepinephrine, dopamine and aldosterone – all markers of unbalanced and excess neurohormonal activity showed a significant reduction upon practising yoga regularly. In other words yoga has the ability to calm down and settle the chaotic activity within your body systems. This seem to have profound healing effects.

Then the researchers studied the physiological parameters of autonomic neurological system's activity. They found out that these subjects showed significant reduction in the resting heart rate, Oxygen consumption, and electrical conducting capacity of the skin – suggesting the quietening of adverse and excess activity of the autonomic neurological function. In addition their breath volume increased – further confirming the improved neurohormonal balance. We already discussed the remarkable benefits of yoga for the diabetic patients. Yoga's effect on reducing blood sugar levels cannot be explained solely by excess calorie expenditure since during yoga you don't burn large quantities of energy. One possible explanation is its ability to restore the hormonal balance that is lost when you develop diabetes. Yoga may well act to increase the levels and the activity of body's natural insulin and decrease the activity of glucagon, the hormone that causes the breakdown of body's energy stores. Such restoration of the neurohormonal balance is also known to bring about protection from coronary heart disease.

Can yoga be used to treat heart disease?

We examined how yoga helps in controlling the risk factors for heart disease and helps prevent heart disease. Scientists and doctors have also demonstrated that by practicing yoga can reduce the blockages in coronary arteries as seen by angiography. Yoga could heal coronary artery disease. They further reported that those patients that practiced yoga had fewer angina episodes and they could exert more physical effort without getting debilitating angina.

The remarkable beneficial effect of yoga on the cholesterol plaques in the coronary arteries was a puzzling observation. One can argue that the effect on your body of practicing yoga may be similar in nature to the remarkable group of wonder drugs called “statins” that are used to treat high cholesterol levels. Statin drugs too act to reduce blood cholesterol levels and at times cause the regression of cholesterol plaques in your arteries. Statins have been shown to increase the production of nitric oxide in the inner lining of arteries. Nitric oxide has very beneficial effects in that it causes enlargement of the narrowed arteries thus facilitating better blood flow. In addition it prevents the build up of cholesterol plaques, prevent smooth muscle cell proliferation and adhesion of white blood cells to the inner lining of the artery – all factors that contribute to coronary heart disease. Especially the latter two factors too are known to contribute to the plaque build up in a direct manner.

Increased activity of the platelets in your blood cause unwanted blood clots to form in your arteries. Such clots when formed within the coronary arteries trigger heart attacks. Statins are known to inhibit the generation of certain chemical agent that enhances platelet activity. Yoga too may be acting in a parallel manner to the statins in that the net effect of yoga is so similar to that of the statins.

Yoga can help accelerate recovery from heart attacks

Yoga has shown to be very beneficial in the recovery process after a heart attack. Practice of yoga improved sleep, appetite, general well being and decreased anxiety among a group of patients who practiced yoga under supervision after a heart attack. In a separate study heart attack patients who practiced *pranayama* yoga breathing showed a rapid improvement in the ability to perform gradually incremental physical tasks. They showed less evidence of fatigue and their efficiency of oxygen use was much superior. Practicing yoga for an year gave better improvements in physical and cardiovascular endurance than conventional aerobic exercise. The yogic practitioners could perform harder physical tasks for longer durations than the control group.

Yoga in heart failure

Researchers also tested the benefits of yoga training to the heart failure patient. Increased and unbalances activity of certain autonomic neurological activity has been associated with the worsening of heart failure. Such adverse autonomic neurological activity increases the mortality of these patients. Drugs that control the excess activity of these neurological elements called "beta blockers" have been shown to improve the symptoms and decrease mortality in heart failure patients. The physiological effects of the practice of yoga seem parallel that of beta-blockers in your body according to scientific findings. Yoga just like beta-blockers can control your heart rate. The other beneficial effects that beta-blockers bring to the heart failure patient were seen with yoga training too.

Under experimental conditions yoga practitioners could tolerate lack of oxygen much better than those that did not practice yoga. Usually under stressful circumstances such as lack of oxygen your autonomic neurological activity, (particularly the so-called "sympathetic" activity) increases setting off the "fight or flight" reaction. This is akin to a panic reaction. But those that practiced yoga showed a blunting of the sympathetic response to the stress created by lack of oxygen. They could make better use of the available oxygen through the practice of yoga breathing. Thus despite lack of availability of oxygen, their blood levels of oxygen remained high when tested. A state of low oxygenation of the blood exists in severe heart failure too. This makes heart failure worse and accelerates death. By practicing yoga breathing heart failure patients can improve their oxygen utilization. The net effect of yoga practice can improve symptoms and prolong life expectancy in heart failure patients.

Yoga for better quality of life

The physical and mental impact of any illness can significantly compromise the quality of your life. This is particularly so with the debilitating and deadly conditions of your heart. Rehabilitation of the cardiac patient also involves helping to improve the quality of life of the patient. In one study conducted to assess the impact of yoga in the improvement of the quality of life of cardiac patients a marked improvement was seen in those that did yoga. This finding was confirmed by performing standard inventory tests that quantify your sense of well-being.

Are there any risks?

Yoga is largely a very safe mode of exercise. Significant fluctuations in the heart rate and blood pressure seen with other more conventional forms of exercise are not seen with yoga due to more controlled and slow nature of its movements. In addition because there is no significant energy burnout and heat generation, yoga does not predispose you to temperature vicissitudes or dehydration. There have been very few reports of muscle, bone or joint injury with yoga practice. There has been only one report in the medical literature so far of any serious injury due to yoga. This was of a stroke suffered by a female yoga practitioner after adopting an unusual neck posture. This incident highlights the fact that nothing is perfectly safe. Therefore caution should be exercise even with very safe practices such as yoga. It is highly recommended that when you start yoga it be done under the guidance and the supervision of an experienced and qualified yoga teacher.

A practical note

There is overwhelming scientific evidence to support the very beneficial effects of yoga in promoting and restoring cardiac health. Similar proof is available to its benefits in other areas of general health and well-being. However, yoga should always be utilized as a complementary means to the more conventional practices of health promotion and treatment of disease. Practice of yoga postures, breathing techniques and meditation may indeed restore your physical health as well as mental well-being.

The best way to start on a yoga program is by finding out more about yoga and increasing your knowledge on the subject. This chapter should have laid a sound scientific foundation to your quest for knowledge on yoga. You should look for a qualified and experienced yoga teacher in your area. Then discuss in detail your expectations and your current health condition with the yoga instructor. Thereafter a suitable yoga program can be embarked on under the supervision and the guidance of your new yoga teacher. Following is an example of some yoga practices that you can try out in consultation with your instructor. These practices have been tested scientifically for their safety and benefits for heart health.

Recommended yoga schedule

1. Yoga breathing:

Uggayi – very slow (3-4 times/min) rhythmical breathing with retention of breath in each cycle. Practice for 10 minutes a day at least. Practice twice a day sitting in the *padmasana* posture and with meditational focus on your breathing. You can also focus on the centre of your forehead with eyes softly closed (the location of the so called "third eye").

2. Body postures

Each of the following postures is to be maintained for 10-20 yoga breaths. Once you have adopted the posture, you should exercise mental concentration by focusing on your breathing or on the center of your forehead –

Shavasana (corpse posture – relaxation pose), Padmasana (Lotus posture), Bhujangasana (Cobra pose), Matsyasana (Fish pose), Ardh-Matsyaendrasana (Spine-twist pose), Yogasana (Yoga pose), Mayurasana (Peacock pose), Imhasana (Lion pose), Gomukhasana (Cow head pose), Sarvangasana (Head down-body up tilt) - your yoga instructor may show you how to adopt each of the above postures. Standard popular books on yoga too may be of help, but the guidance of a qualified teacher or guru is of prime importance.

Practice the above postures for a total of 40-60 minutes each day or as often as possible. It is easier and better to develop a certain routine by setting apart some quiet moments in your day to practice yoga in a setting of total relaxation, leisure and tranquility. At the end of the session adopt the Shavasana pose for a period of fifteen minutes or as long as you can afford. As you lie on the matt in this posture voluntarily let different parts of your body be put in to total limp-relaxation. You should do this in a sequential manner starting from the head all the way to your toes. You should make every muscle in your body flaccid and lifelessly relaxed. This form of voluntary relaxation should relax your body in a similar manner to its relaxation during the deep phase (the REM phase) of your sleep cycle. At the end of the session itself you may start to feel the deep sense of total body and mind relaxation, refreshment and renewal. In the long term, as you practice yoga regularly you may feel the gradual transformation within your self. You may feel fresh and energetic and free of stress constantly. Your doctor should be informed about your commencing yoga exercises if you have been diagnosed with heart disease. As you practice yoga, your doctor too may notice the positive changes in your physiological parameters such your pulse rate, blood pressure and body mass index etc.

Tai Chi and heart health

Tai Chi is an ancient Chinese tradition of physical exercise. It has two basic components. The first involves the synchronized and coordinated rhythmic body movements. The second is mental concentration in the form of meditation. The practice of Tai Chi was originally developed by the Chinese Taoist martial artists and traditional Chinese physicians. Practice of Tai Chi also has a strong philosophical basis according to the experts. According to this ancient philosophy the practice of Tai Chi involves the generation and the promotion of "internal energy" within your self. This process is represented by the word "Chi". Just like yoga Tai Chi too derives its healing properties through the restoration of the strong wholesome interrelationship between mental and physical faculties of your body. The practice of Tai Chi is very prevalent in China and also among the Chinese living all over the world. It has been identified as an integral part of the traditional Chinese lifestyle. By practicing Tai Chi you tune in to the natural balance of your self, first physically and then mentally. Its practice has been described as being profoundly relaxing, refreshing and relieving.

There are different forms and traditions of Tai Chi techniques. But there is uniformity in the general principles of its practice. As a form of exercise and recreation it is fast becoming popular in the west. Tai Chi has already been incorporated to the practice of rehabilitation in various medical specialties including geriatrics and cardiology. Much attention has been paid by the scientific community to studying the health benefits of Tai Chi lately. Most convincing evidence to the benefits of Tai Chi in the management of patients comes from the studies done among the elderly patients. Tai Chi has demonstrated to be particularly effective in enhancing the balance and body awareness. This effect is brought about by the performance of slow, graceful, and precise body movements. In the elderly practice of Tai Chi has been effective in preventing falls through the restoration of balance. It is also found out to be able to significantly cut the risk of falls among older people. It also help improve muscular strength. Another significant fact that came to light through these studies was the that adoption of relatively low tech, traditional methods may bring benefits that far exceed those from more sophisticated methods and interventions and in the process save millions of dollars to the healthcare budget. Research has also demonstrated the beneficial effect that can be obtained from the practice of Tai Chi particularly in heart disease. These benefits seem to go way beyond the simple improvement of balance and coordination.

Tai Chi technique involves slow continuous movements that bring about a smooth transition of different body postures. In addition Tai Chi also involves controlled breathing exercises. It helps to improve balance and coordination. It is also known to be beneficial in improving physical and mental health. Tai Chi may well correct the neurohormonal imbalances in your body thus promoting health.

Researchers have found out that practicing Tai Chi helped patients who had heart attacks to recover faster. Patients are prescribed drugs to slow their heart rate after a heart attack. This effect of slowing the heart rate was also brought about by the practice of Tai Chi. Tai Chi can also effectively reduce blood pressure in patients suffering from high blood pressure. Researchers have shown that the blood pressure lowering effect of Tai Chi is much stronger than the blood pressure lowering effect of aerobic exercise. Patients who were not fit or strong enough to perform low intensity aerobic exercise after a heart attack could still perform the slow and gentle movements of Tai Chi.

Long term practice of Tai Chi seems to improve the body's ability to extract oxygen from the air. This is an index of physical fitness. Doctors studying those who practiced Tai Chi observed that their age related decline in physical fitness and capacity to extract oxygen from air slowed down. Thus in a way Tai Chi slowed down the process of aging.

A major challenge in exercise programs for heart patients is their high drop out rates. But it has been observed that the programs for heart patients that had Tai Chi incorporated as a major component had less numbers dropping out. Increasingly more and more cardiac rehabilitation facilities in big hospitals in the west are incorporating Tai Chi into their rehabilitation programs. Surveys have revealed that most cardiac rehabilitation facilities have a keen interest in incorporating Tai Chi into their regular practice and service. Lack of funding and expertise have been identified as impediments against more wide spread use of this exercise modality. According to scientific literature practice of Tai Chi can also prolong life in the older individuals.

Another major benefit of Tai Chi is its safety. The gentle smooth movements put minimal strain on the joints and muscles thus preventing injury to the same. It does not cause rapid increases in the blood pressure and the heart rate and therefore does not put the heart and the circulatory system under excessive strain. This is particularly important in the elderly and the physically weak heart patients.

Tai Chi can be optimal for the more physically fit and the younger individuals who desire a more strenuous physical workout too. It has been demonstrated that by the changing the technique of practice Tai Chi can exercise the heart as much as aerobic exercise does. Such technical changes include deeper stances, movement against resistance and movement at a faster pace. Performed thus Tai Chi is converted to a form of aerobic exercise.

Physical and mental effects of the practice of Tai Chi has a very important stress relieving aspects too according to the experts. This can be demonstrated in the slowing of heart rate, slowing of breathing and the improved general sense of well being observed in those who practice this art. This may be of great benefit to heart health. Type A personality that is described as being highly stressed and the type D personality that is described as being highly anxious have been related to heart disease as certain risk factors. Stress relieving effect of Tai Chi may address this risk factor that is otherwise hard to modify in the very fast paced and competitive modern day lifestyle. The popularity of Tai Chi may due to several factors that include its convenience of practice. It is economical in that no specialized equipment or settings are needed. Tai Chi can be practiced any where there is enough space to move the body by few steps to each side.

How to start Tai Chi

The best way to start practicing Tai Chi is by joining a local group that offers group lessons under an expert instructor. As with any form of physical exercise before commencing you should discuss it with your doctor. Even your doctor may help you find a recommendable Tai Chi teacher or a group. Tai Chi can be incorporated in to your life style once mastered.

Tai Chi is a very convenient form of exercise. Only ten to fifteen minutes' of exercise may be all that is needed for a complete session. Thus it rarely necessitate rearranging of schedules or setting apart hours for physical exercise. Tai Chi has very important economic conveniences too. As far as infrastructure is concerned, you can practice Tai Chi in you office, bedroom, TV lounge, garden or even the public park. Tai Chi does not require special gear. All you need is comfortable clothing such as a sweat-absorbing top, a pair of loose fitting pants and comfortable foot wear with flat soles.

Pilates

Pilates is a form of alternative exercise that is becoming increasingly popular since of late. It was initially introduced by Joseph Pilates an American physical therapist of German origin. Pilates too just like yoga and Tai Chi focuses on body movements coupled with emphasis on mental concentration. In addition it has much focus on controlled breathing techniques and postural correction. Body movements of Pilates exercise are smooth and slow. Experts define these movements as smooth transitions of different postures in one continuum. Benefits attributed to regular practice of Pilates include weight loss, improvement of posture, improved flexibility and mental and physical relaxation. An important feature of Pilates is the relative safety from injury because of the low impact nature of the involved movements.

Pilates has not been subjected to scientific experimentation in the setting of health promotion as yoga or Tai Chi. However practitioners that include many high profile public figures claim significant benefits and attribute their good health and feeling of well being to the regular practice of Pilates. The sheer nature of the methods and techniques and the movements suggest it to be similar to yoga and Tai Chi. Therefore one can assume the benefits for cardiac health as well as general health to be similar in nature.

Pilates can be practiced with minimum of facilities, equipment or gear. Advanced techniques may need certain equipment that still can be provided without too much of a cost. The many practitioners of the technique include people of all walks of life, of all ages and of different levels of physical fitness. Many practitioners and experts in the field promote Pilates as an ideal form of exercise to be incorporated in the setting of cardiac disease prevention and rehabilitation.

Chapter 12

Tuning in: A Road Map to Life

Creating the right balance between the body functions and mind functions is the key to greater health and vitality. As we have learned and experienced from reading this book, heart disease is caused by the adverse effects of certain risk factors affecting the proper and normal functioning of your body systems. These adverse effects start their activity in the very microscopic- cellular level in your body. For example toxic and harmful effects of bad cholesterol are first seen at the molecular level with its oxidation and at cellular level with its attacking and damaging of the single cell layer that makes up your endothelium. In a similar manner, toxic molecules from the cigarette smoke you inhale attack and disrupt the endothelium at the cellular level. These cellular damages evolve and progress to have a collective detrimental effect on your body. These effects transform into heart disease. Further progression of it can lead to irreversible organ damage (heart attacks, heart failure etc.) and even death.

The real face of mind-body medicine or holistic health is best evident at the cellular level in your body. The most scientific explanation to this phenomenon can be found there and the evidence to its importance is irrefutable. At this cellular level your body and mind becomes one single entity. At this ultramicroscopic level your mind and your body have no separate identities or divisions. In one sense it parallels the unified theory of matter and energy. At the level of sub atomic particles or quantum's there is no separation of matter and energy. Matter is energy and energy is matter and they exist in an interchanging equilibrium. Disruption of this balance creates catastrophe and leads to energy release of fission and fusion. In a similar manner at the cellular level your body is mind and your mind is body, existing in equilibrium.

At this level the mind and the body operate in synchrony. As the structures get larger you appreciate the division between the body and the mind more and more. At the cellular level the functions are mediated and controlled by chemical compounds that act as messengers. These messengers are called neurochemicals, neurohormones or neuropeptides. These same chemical classes act within the brain and the neurological system to relay messages and to bring about our thought, emotional and mental processes. In fact the entire brain and the neurological systems are made up of such chemical constituents.

It is at this level that the mind influences your body and the body influences your mind in a profound way. It is so profound that your functioning as a being is dependent on what happens at this level. The disruption of this balance leads to ill health of mind or body.
So to rectify the issues related to your body's health, the resources of your mind should be harnessed in the proper manner. In a similar manner for your mind 's health the resources of your body should be harnessed correctly. The body mind relationship or the balance is an interrelated, interdependent, dichotomous phenomenon. The choices you make each day with regards to your life style have a great impact on the mind-body balance and thus on your health. Tuning into this mind body balance and restoring imbalances are the essences of healthy living. I will introduce you to this wonderful world of your inner (cellular) being and teach you the methods by which you may maintain the wholesome balance in the unified mind-body system.

Revitalize your mind

First step to right living is revitalizing and restoring the mind factors in your being. Knowledge, contemplation (meditation or focus) and right thinking are the three key elements of the wholesome mind factor.

Knowledge

This book attempted to provide you with the all-important knowledge related to heart disease and heart health. In addition it provided you with the knowledge on the Eastern philosophy related to heart health and general health and well-being. To understand the important practical applications of mind body techniques, knowledge of the ancient Indian medical tradition of Ayurveda is very important. Different elements we discussed in the relevant chapters of this book such as yoga are derivatives of this vast health related philosophy that has been identified as one of the most profound and time tested methods of integrated mind-body medical systems in the world.

Knowledge is awareness. The more you know the truth about your body and you mind the more power you have over these elements. Knowledge on the key areas of heart disease and heart health gives you a certain grasp or control over issues related to your heart health. Learning about what preventive means and therapeutic means available against heart disease enables you to make powerful and wise choices related to your own well being. The knowledge on the background of the therapies (how treatment forms are developed and how they act etc.) available today gives you further confidence when it comes to discussing your options with your doctor and making right consensual choices. Knowledge of nutrition and diet gives you the power of choice when it comes to what you eat. Thus you may eat only what is safe and wholesome.

Focus

Second principle element of the mind factor is the conscious attempts at focusing your thoughts and purifying your mind of the unnecessary information that may create confusion and turmoil within your mind. The objective is to create a sound, clear and peaceful mind. A mind of clarity and tranquility that is fresh and stable. When the mind is rested thus, the wholesome neurochemical balances are restored. This restored balance lays the foundation of good health within you. This is achieved by meditation and thought control. This way you master your mind and the mind shall master your body function, bringing you the benefits of good health and vitality. In the chapter on yoga I repeatedly showed you the amazing impact the mindfulness-based practices have on the physiological functions of your body such as the blood pressure, heart rate, lung function and even the levels of different chemical constituents in your blood.

Just like meditation prayer is a very a powerful means by which you can control your body functions to effect healing. There is increased emphasis placed on prayer among the general public for the purpose of healing and preservation of good health. Surveys have revealed that prayers are on most occasion made for health and healing. And the effects and the power of prayer have been scientifically proven. Furthermore the most convincing and dramatic stories to the proof of its power are in the individual experiences of miracles and restoration. Prayer gives you freedom from depression and anxiety. It gives you power.

It has been a well-known fact in the medical circles that those who attend church regularly had very low incidence of heart disease and mental disorders. In head to head comparisons those who consistently attend church or belonged to highly spiritual faith groups lived the healthiest and longest lives. Through prayer you make a journey to be in oneness with your Creator that is the essence of your inner being and your spirituality. This inward journey is meant to empower, energize and revitalize your whole being.

Thinking

The third element of your mind factor is right thinking. This is the practical and outward expression of your mind function. This involves analytical ability, insight, vision and resolve. The results of thinking are your choices. You are what you think you are. Your thought processes decide your destiny including the destiny of your health. Right thinking is based on the status of your mind and the level of your knowledge (the previous two elements discussed above). Always think right and positive. Have a positive desire. A positive attitude is the first step to good health. No matter what your circumstances are you should first think within your self that you choose health. Attaining good health should be your one resolve.

Remember good health is not a privilege but a choice.

Thought purification has amazing healing properties. It is imperative that you think right of your own self. This should enhance your self-image and establish within you an absolute sense of self worth. You are special, unique and precious. You have the control over your destiny. You are very special and important. Your choices do matter. Then think right about others and your environment. Make it a goal of your life to give, love and serve. Each day strive to make somebody else happy, in that process you may find happiness for yourself. This happiness will be free of fear or anxiety. Thus the neuro-chemical system and the hormonal system of your body (which are the material expressions of your mind) may function in the right balance thus avoiding the build up of adverse chemical secretions that can cause harm to your organs, particularly your heart.

Another important aspect of thinking right involves developing a passion for living. Dream big, develop visions and have goals in life that you would want to work at with all your heart. Be thankful for each day.

The combination

When you are reconditioned by knowledge and motivated by mental mastery, the application of healthy living principles becomes a natural process for you. This application is reflected in your daily choices and your life style. It all involves making wise and well balanced choices. With mental mastery and spiritual strength you can control your proclivity to make unhealthy and bad choices. It gives you the power to resist unhealthy and extreme indulgences. It helps you to make right choices regarding your life style, spiritual practices, diet, physical activity, recreation etc.

Always be conscious of the three fundamental mind factors of your being. Strive to attain self-mastery through the development of your knowledge, mental focus and right thinking. These factors may restore and put right the mind factor of your health. At all times think within your self whether you know enough about anything and everything that concerns you. Keep your mind clear and sound through constant meditation or prayer. Then when it comes to lifestyle and daily living ask your self constantly whether you are making the right choices. Right choices are that which will not harm your body and your mind but contribute to its wellness.

Exercises to keep your mind factors sound

1. Enhance your knowledge: Read, study, listen and inquire about how your body and mind functions, how diseases develop, how they are treated, how these treatment techniques are developed, and how disease could be prevented. Knowledge gives you a stable and sound foundation to the building up of your healthy lifestyle. Be on a journey of discovery constantly. Remember knowledge is power and the power shall set you free!

2. Learn a meditation technique: yoga meditation is ideal in this regard because it had been scientifically proven, it is user friendly and very effective.

3. Pray and keep your mind clean and powerful. The healing power of prayer too is scientifically proven.

4. Think right, and about good and positive things. Thus you constantly purify your mind. This purification cleanses body function starting from the cellular level. This will purify your internal body systems and restore and preserve health.

5. Practice honesty, humility, love, compassion, peace, sacrificial giving and other virtuous acts – you may be amazed by the positive mental effects you get from the practice of such thoughts in your mind.

Mind-body applications for heath and complete self renewal

You are defined by your choices. Health is no exception. You will be healthy only if you choose to be healthy. The choices you make are the material expressions of your mind factors. Once you have put right your mind factors using the three keys that I have given to you in the previous section of this chapter, you are ready to make practical applications of it for your new healthy life style.

Practice hygiene

Make cleanliness a habit. Cleanliness of the outside of your body as well as the inside of your body is important to preserve good heart health. Personal hygiene is the result of outward cleanliness. Cleanliness inside of your body starts at the very cellular level. Purification of you internal body systems starting from the cellular level to the level of your whole being involves eating right, drinking right, sleeping right, physical exercising and medicating right (if necessary). Body hygiene and internal body system purity go hand in hand.

Breath right

Be conscious of you breathing. This is what keeps you alive every moment of your life. Breath right – Whenever possible for a moment practice *"pranayama"* or equivalent breathing. This can be done at any time anywhere. Recital of the *manthra "om"* as in yoga practice or the recital of the Holy Rosary as per the practice of the Catholics too is equivalent to *"pranayama"*. This helps to restore your body's baroreflex sensitivity and heart rate variability, two major requirements for cardiovascular health. This too will readjust your neurological and hormonal balance to the optimal. Practicing this at instances of high stress will not only relieve stress but also prevent the effects of the stressful situation affecting your health and damaging your body. This type of breathing should bring down the rate of breathing to 6 breaths per minute.

Eat right

Eating in moderation with the awareness of what you eat and how much you eat is the key to eating right. You should know your objective of eating right. First and foremost it is to ensure good health and preserve your heart. Losing weight and controlling other cardiac risk factors through diet is fundamental in this regard. As we have discussed in this book earlier I advocate constant practice of food watching and portion control as the best strategy for healthy eating. Know what you eat and choose what is good. Do not let your eyes or your tongue rule your eating habits. Rather let your well informed and well-focused mind do it. Eat small portions that are enough to satisfy your hunger. Let the predominant part of your diet be fresh vegetables, fresh fruits, nuts and legumes. Eat less calories than you need for your daily activities. Try to generate the cleansing habit of fasting or skipping two or more meals at least once a month. This may be a stressful exercise at first. But as you persevere you may experience a deep sense of fulfillment and satisfaction out of fasting. Remember also to have your glass of red wine each day–just one glass, no more and no less!

At the start of the day drink a full glass of water with a drop of pure bee's honey dissolved in it, into an empty stomach. This ancient practice of some parts of India is known to confer good health and longevity. While no scientific studies have been carried out to verify its efficacy, over five thousand years of anecdotal evidence is hard to ignore.
The lessons on eating right are further reviewed later in this chapter in the introduction to the remarkable "life diet".

Exercise right

Heart disease is a result of bad lifestyle. This is the lifestyle of over eating and physical inactivity. To liberate yourself from the imprisonment of this sorry life style get your mind factors to make you active. Start with some form of physical activity, like walking.

Do it daily at least for half an hour. As you develop the three mind factors to act you will be motivated to do more exercise with a purpose and a passion. Diversify the type of exercises you do to make it more enjoyable. Jogging, swimming, golf and cycling would be the next step up. Become obsessive about doing your daily session of exercise. Make it a part of your life style. Gradually get serious about your exercising. Join a gym, hire a personal trainer, buy new exercise equipment thus make investments of money, time and commitment to your exercise program.

Make sure you have discussed with your doctor prior to commencing exercise if you are over the age of forty. Remember to warm up and warm down before and after exercise sessions. You may see yourself improving as you go along with your new habit. You will start to look and feel younger. You will feel the constant burst of energy and vitality. You will start to lose weight and look good. All these results will motivate you even more to persist with your exercising.

Now that you also know the benefits of alternative forms of exercise, commence yoga, Tai Chi or pilates. Look for a local yoga class and start doing yoga regularly. Yoga will activate that vital connection between your mind and your body. You will start to feel the freshness in your everyday life. Your life will become a new experience. You will see life as a new discovery and a new passion each passing day.

Exercising regularly would mean also being physically active with everything and every aspect in your life. Avoid the elevator and take the stairs. Take strolls to your short distance destinations and avoid driving. Develop a desire to be physically more active at every opportunity. When you do this your doctor too may observe the transformation in your health. Your blood pressure, cholesterol level, blood sugar level and even the mental state would show improvements. Such developments may be so dramatic at times that your doctor may even consider reducing the amount of medications you take.

Medicate right

Though synthetic and fraught with side effects medications are not all bad news! All medications the doctors give you may be important for your health. Therefore it is important that you ensure 100% compliance. But you may also be taking unnecessary medications, doctor given or self initiated. Your doctor may review the need for some medications as your body functions get better with the practice of your good mind body techniques. Always be guided by your doctor because he is responsible for your health. But this should no longer be blind following because you have acquired enough knowledge to be able to actively participate in the crucial decision making process with regards to your life and your health. Now it is a collective responsibility of yours and your doctor's. You may benefit from the wonder drug statin. Talk to your doctor. Even if your cholesterol is normal you may find benefits in the long run. It works to put right the all-important neurochemicals at the cellular level. Statins act like mind-body pep pills. Stains have demonstrated convincing life saving benefits far and beyond simple cholesterol reduction.

Another drug that you may benefit from is aspirin. Aspirin help to keep your blood thin thus preventing unnecessary clots that cause heart attacks and strokes from forming in your circulation. Aspirin also acts at the cellular level to reduce the activity of neurochemicals that mediate inflammation and thus disease. This very cheap drug has shown life saving and disease preventing benefits. Check with your doctor to see whether you too should be on aspirin.

Discoveries of modern medicine are truly amazing and most such advanced medical care is available widely to everyone. It is your doctor that would facilitate the use of this marvelous resource to help you live a healthy life. Statin drugs and aspirin have become the corner stones of modern day preventive treatment of cardiovascular disease.
In addition if you have a heart condition that need treatment, it is

important that you comply with all the drugs you have been prescribed by your doctor. Most drugs used today have proven life saving values and safety records. As you practice the mind-body principles you learned from this book and apply the healthy living principles to your life, your doctor may reduce your dependence on medications by dose reduction and reduction of the number of drugs you have to take on a regular basis.

Giving up addictions

As you practice the mind-body techniques you may find it easy to give up your harmful habits of substance dependence such as smoking, excess alcohol consumption and narcotic abuse. It is an absolute requirement for good health that you do away with any form of substance abuse. Knowledge, focus and thinking, the three keys of the sound mind factor will help you give up your addictions, if you practice these principles with passion and serious effort. First you should make a concrete resolve to stop your harmful habit. Then stop it abruptly once and for all. Research has shown that the best way to stop a harmful habit is to go cold turkey and recover from the withdrawals. Once you overcome the short-term effects of the withdrawal symptoms and the cravings you will be completely free of your addiction. The mind body practices you learn from this book will help you to be strong against the withdrawal symptoms and the cravings. This works wonders compared to attempting to give up gradually.

Recreation and rest

Do things for enjoyment. Life is to be enjoyed, not endured. Develop an appreciation for the finer things in life. Listen to healing and relaxing music. Appreciate art. Be passionate about making love to your significant other. Scientific research has shown that married people live longer and among the married those that have sex more live longer.
Sleep well. Over sleeping is as harmful as sleep deprivation.

Research has shown that those who sleep moderately, about six hours each 24 hours live the longest.

The Life Diet

There are many diets out there and each has a certain objective. Most of the popular diets seem to be very effective in bringing about the desired changes. Most of the diets are aimed at bringing about weight loss. Other diets are meant to control blood sugar levels in the diabetics and lower cholesterol in those with high cholesterol levels. In addition diet gurus and experts in alternative medicine have formulated diets to cleanse different body organs and these too seem to make people feel good once adopted.

The effect and efficiency of the diabetic diets and the low cholesterol diets can be tested by testing blood for sugar levels or the cholesterol levels respectively after the recommended period and also by monitoring blood levels at constant intervals. The efficacy of the weight loss diets too can be observed by monitoring body weight while being on the diet. The efficacy of many other diets can only be measured through the evaluation of the level of your subjective well-being. That is by assessing how the person who is on the diet feels generally. Thus it is evident that apart from the disease specific diets and weight loss diets, the other special diets can hardly be scientifically tested. However anecdotal evidence and theoretical possibilities may justify such diets.

The heart healthy "life diet" I introduce in this book is aimed at controlling coronary risk factors and thus promoting health. It is based on firm scientific evidence to the efficacy of the fundamental principles on which it is based. Among the many diets that have been recommended and suggested for the promotion of cardiac health only the "Mediterranean diet" and the "Indo-Mediterranean diet" have come out as being effective at decreasing the incidence of heart attacks and prolonging life expectancy.

You may remember the Mediterranean diet and the Indo-Mediterranean diet that I introduced to you in the chapter on diet and nutrition previously. I may reinforce your knowledge on these diets as building your mind factor of knowledge may help you in the practical application of the ideal diet principles. Scientists have long observed that people living in the Mediterranean region had a very low incidence of heart disease. In addition their coronary risk factors such as high blood pressure, diabetes and cholesterol levels too were not as high as it is elsewhere in the western world. Scientists attributed this health effects to the traditional Mediterranean diet and tested this hypothesis by comparing people who were maintained on the Mediterranean diet with control populations maintained on standard western diet. The tests showed that the Mediterranean diet was very effective in controlling coronary risk factors, reducing the incidence of heart disease and preventing premature deaths due to heart attacks.

A study called the "*Seven countries study*" conducted in the 1950s showed that people in the island of Crete and Greece had low incidence of heart disease and certain cancers and had a long life expectancy despite eating food high in fats. Their traditional diet was identified as the reason for these health benefits. The main feature of this diet was the high content of plant foods such as vegetables, fruits, whole grain cereals, nuts and legumes. Their main source of fat was from olive oil. The diet included some fish and poultry. However it had very low levels of red meat. Another important ingredient of this diet was wine that was mostly consumed in strict moderation with the meals.

The first clinical evidence of the benefits of the Mediterranean diet was demonstrated in the *Lyon Diet Study* of which the results were published in the medical journal Lancet in 1994. In this study the researchers showed that those who consumed the Mediterranean diet had a 73% reduction in the rates of heart disease and a 70% reduction in the mortality rates after a period of just over 2 years. In a study published recently in the New England Journal of Medicine involving over 20,000 subjects a group of scientists led by Trichopoulou showed that adherence to the traditional Mediterranean diet could significantly lower the rates of heart disease, certain cancers and overall mortality. They also showed that the effect of the diet was not due to a single ingredient or a component of the diet but the result of the cumulative and collective effect of all the ingredients.

In 2002 a group of scientists led by Singh introduced the concept of the Indo-Mediterranean diet that lowered the rates of fatal heart attacks and sudden death due to heart disease by significant proportions. These facts were demonstrated in a study conducted involving 1000 patients with already diagnosed heart disease or who were at a high risk of coronary artery disease unlike the study involving the Mediterranean diet where all participants were healthy. The remarkable results of this study too were published in the Lancet. The Indo-Mediterranean diet had high levels of mustard or soybean oil, nuts, vegetables, fruits and whole grains.

Anecdotal evidence and evidence from large population based studies from some rural areas of the far-east (China, Korea and Japan) report very low incidence of heart disease and cancers and longevity. While many environmental factors may contribute to this, their diet too is considered to play an integral role. What is more interesting is that despite the regions being diverse, vast and inhabited by over a billion people their dietary habits have some fundamental commonalities. Once again we see the trend repeated. Their diet, just like the Mediterranean diet and the Indo-Mediterranean diet has high levels of vegetables, fruits, nuts and whole grain. In addition sea-weeds and soy products are featured dominantly in the far-eastern diet. Instead of wine as in the Mediterranean diet, the Far Eastern diet features the consumption of large amounts of tea. Another important aspect of the Far Eastern diet is the high level of fish consumption, low to moderate levels of poultry consumption and near zero consumption of red meats.

Among the populations studied in the different diet forms discussed above, outside the Mediterranean region obesity was practically unheard of in the other regions. And the Indian and the Far Eastern regions are comprised of over two billion people- more than two third of the world's population! What is the significant difference between the dietary habits of the Far East and the South Asian regions that was different to that of the Mediterranean belt? Yes it is the proportion of fat in the meal and portion size. While in the

Mediterranean region there is high consumption of fat and the portion size of each meal is large, in the Asian regions the fat content is low and the portion size is much smaller.

A combination of the Indo-Mediterranean or Far Eastern diet with low fat content, controlled carbohydrate content and portion control seem ideal for good health, longevity and importantly weight control. So what is this "life saving and figure friendly diet"? The above evidence makes the answer to this important question quite simple and very straight-forward. Eat more vegetables, fruits, nuts, legumes (including soy beans), mono/unsaturated fats, small quantities of alcohol, tea and consume smaller portions of meals just adequate to satisfy your hunger. These are the key aspects of the "Life Diet". Given the vast array of different food types incorporated to the definition, the variety is not restrictive at all. So it is not a boring diet – but a very diverse and exciting diet. It is never bland, but rich in taste and flavor. The fundamental ingredients of the ideal diet or the "Life-Diet" are as follows:

-Mono unsaturated/ poly-unsaturated fats (olive oil, Canola oil, soy bean oil)
-Unprocessed / whole grain carbohydrates (thus carbohydrates with a low glycemic index)
-Fresh vegetables and those with high content of fiber
-Green leafy vegetables
-Fresh fruits
-Nuts and legumes
-Soy products
-Seafood/ fish
-Low to moderate levels of poultry
-Low or no red meats
-Smaller portions of meals with low fat content
-Small amount of alcohol with meals
-Large quantities of tea
-A day of fasting (for about 18 hours: start at midnight and end at 6 pm the following evening) at regular intervals (monthly to start with)

The above dietary model is the basis of the "Life Diet" – while this diet gives you longevity it also lets you live to the max each day – enjoy your meals, be healthy and be slim. Add to this moderate level physical activity and mind-body exercise (yoga, meditation, *pranayama* breathing) – you got the plan for ideal living. Develop the right attitude- we all can make the world a better place!

In formulating the concept of the "Life Diet" I attempted to make wise eating simple. While there is great value in carb counting, calorie counting and fat estimating, there is an inherent complexity in performing the same every time you eat something. Thus precise measurement of these factors in your diet makes healthy eating burdensome. In the "Life Diet" model I introduce choosing the right food types with some pre-knowledge (as provided in this book) and consuming limited portion sizes without having to worry about the precise measurement of the dietary constituents.

Practical tips for the "Life Diet"

1. Your total daily fat consumption should be less than 30% of your daily calorie intake.
2. Your total daily calorie intake should be less than 2000 kilocalories for females and less than 2500 kilocalories for males.
3. When the daily calorie in take is 2000-2500, your total daily fat intake should be less than 65 grams/ your total saturated fat intake should be less than 20 grams.
4. Avoid any food that is braised, fried or basted that has high levels of fat. Au gratin or crispy food too has high fat content.
5. Avoid or minimize food containing hydrogenated oils, partially hydrogenated oils and vegetable shortening-they are high in trans fats. Use low fat mayonnaise and salad dressings made of the same. Choose low fat salad dressings when going for prepared dressings.
6. Balsamic vinegar is a healthy alternative to salad dressing
7. Eat more vegetarian meals or fish. When eating meat choose lean cuts.
8. Eat food high in fiber, eg: celery, bran. Aim to eat more than 40g of fiber each day.

9. Limit the starch and plain carbohydrate content of your food by avoiding bread, cakes, rice, pasta, chocolates, sugar and pastry. Eat salads and fruits. Eat more legumes and soy products. Your total carbohydrate intake should be less than 200 grams each day. Avoid white carbohydrates at all times (white bread, white rice etc.). Eat only the whole-grain carbs, even that in limited quantities.

10. Avoid food with high salt content. Know that food that is pickled, cured, smoked have high levels of sodium. Also broth, soy sauce, MSG, teriyaki sauce and other oriental sauces have high levels of sodium. Ordinary canned food too has high sodium content.

Flavoring stock has high levels of salt. Use herbs and spices instead for flavoring.

11. Very frequently eat meals consisting only of fresh vegetables and fruits – particularly for breakfast and lunch. Add soy products (that contain high levels of isoflavones) and tea to your diet often.

11. The fundamental format of the life diet is quite simple. The basic plan of the "Life Diet" is as follows-

Breakfast – High grain / whole wheat food 1 serving, fruit 1 serving, skim dairy product or equivalent 1 serving, egg white preparation, tea

Lunch – Fresh vegetable with legumes (and fish) salad 1 serving, fresh fruit 1 serving

Dinner – lean meat (preferably white meat or fish) or textured soy protein, vegetables, red or white wine 1 glass, low calorie/non-fat dessert

Between meal snacks are limited to small servings of roasted/ non-salted nuts and fruit slices

Rice (particularly white varieties), white bread, food containing trans fats (pastries, biscuits, cakes, fries etc.), bagel, full cream dairy products, red meats, processed meats, fried foods and sweet desserts are altogether excluded from the "Life Diet". I have presented a selection of suggested daily meal plans according to the above "Life Diet" principle at the end of this chapter. As you become familiar with the dietary concepts introduced in this book and as you practice the "Life Diet" you may be able to prepare your own "Life Diet" meals according to its fundamental principles and the basic patterns.

Tips when choosing meals

Italian

1. Eat less pasta and bread, Order piccata or saltimbocca that have less fat, eat the green salad and ask for fresh chopped tomatoes as against tomato sauce
2. Sautéed portabella mushrooms, salad with parmesan cheese, antipasto, marinated peppers and eggplant parmesan are good
3. Avoid fettuccine Alfredo, risotto and any thing that is fried
4. Ask for roasted fish or grilled seafood
5. Avoid chicken or veal parmesan
6. Stracciatella soup is good.

Chinese

1. Eat steamed or broiled dishes, avoid the fried
2. Avoid salt and sugar rich sauces
3. Avoid fried rice, prawn crackers and fried dim sums
4. Eat steamed tofu or steamed whole fish
5. Avoid noodle dishes and sweet and sour pork
6. Eat Chinese green vegetables and Chinese mushroom
7. Drink plenty of green tea

Thai

1. Thai salads are delicious and healthy

2. Avoid curries cooked in thick coconut milk
3. Ask for grilled meats instead of the fried meats
4. Limit your rice intake
5. Choose fish curries and seafood preparations

Indian

1. Choose salads and vegetarian dishes
2. Avoid fried rice preparations and fried breads such as Poori
3. Channa dhal is good
4. Tandoori is good because it is oven grilled but beware of the salt content
5. Avoid samosa that is very high in carbohydrates
6. Avoid dishes cooked in cream and ghee
7. Avoid fried dishes,

Japanese

1. Avoid Tempura dishes and the other fried preparations
2. Eat the Japanese salad and tofu preparations
3. Ask for sushi with more fish and less rice.
4. Avoid soba and other noodles dishes
5. Limit the soy sauce amount you add to your food
6. Miso soup is good
7. Choose grilled Teppenyaki
8. Drink plenty of green tea

Suggested sample meals

Day 1
Breakfast: Bircher muesli with raisins and nuts, Low fat yogurt, Two slices of cantaloupe, Green or black tea
Lunch: Tuna and pepper salad, banana
Dinner: Poached sea bass, Baked onions, Tossed green salad, Glass of wine, Poached winter fruits for dessert

Day 2
Breakfast: Whole grain toast with olive oil spread, an apple, Swiss oat meal made with non-fat milk, English breakfast tea
Lunch: Lentil salad, Bowl of mixed berries
Dinner: Vegetable antipasto salad, Seafood Paella (made of brown rice) with artichokes, glass of wine, Frozen peach yogurt for dessert

Day 3
Breakfast: Hi fibre- organic muffin, low fat cheese, cup of cherries, green tea
Lunch: Portobello mushrooms stuffed with Spinach and Couscous, dried fruit salad
Dinner: Tomato Bruschetta, Chicken, Tomato and White Bean Penne, Glass of wine, Sweet almond tofu dessert

Day 4
Breakfast: Egg-white omelets with mushroom, non-fat yogurt, a banana, lemon tea
Lunch: Skate salad, tropical fruit selection (unsweetened)
Dinner: Celery root and spinach soup, Pasta con le Sarde (pasta with sardines), glass of wine, Oranges with Tarragon syrup for dessert

Day 5
Breakfast: Two slices of whole grain toast, Toasted muesli with non fat yogurt, Slice of fresh papaya with lime, Earl Grey tea
Lunch: Purslane and spinach salad, Tain of tomatoes and peppers, Orange
Dinner: Raita salad, Masala dosa with alu paneer, Glass of wine, Non-fat kulfi for dessert

Day 6
Breakfast: Egg-white scrambled with fresh tomato, Non-fat banana smoothie with sliced banana, Ceylon tea
Lunch: Red pepper salad with olives and anchovies, Tuna with salsa cruda, Blue berries
Dinner: Shrimp with green sauce, Marsala chicken with fennel, Glass of wine, Strawberry-yogurt mousse for dessert

Day 7

Breakfast: Whole grain sandwich with avocado, bean sprouts and goat cheese, Slice of pineapple, Darjeeling tea

Lunch: Cucumber soup with borage, Fava bean salad with prosciutto, Seedless grapes

Dinner: Grilled baby octopus, Wild salmon steak with tomato and bell pepper salsa, Glass of wine, Pistachio baklava for dessert

Notes